Secrets of Yogic Breathing
Vayu Siddhi

A Guide to Pranayama, Ashtanga
Yoga's Fourth Limb

with David Garrigues

Contents

This book is intended to be used with the video series.

Acknowledgments

Thank you, Joy Marzec, for being with me all the way through the *Vayu Siddhi* video series/book project from its rather perilous beginning to completion. The idea to offer these teachings on pranayama was born when we were rendered immovable by the Great Spirit during our visit to the Andaman Islands off the coast of India in 2010. During our month stay an extremely intense back spasm left me with only a breathing practice and a lot free time. This book is the fruit of the seeds that were planted within me during that enforced breathing intensive. Without your help from then until now there would be no book.

Thanks to Joanna Darlington for her dedication in helping me share my teachings and her tireless, careful work, and meticulous attention to detail in editing and assembling this book. Thanks to Natasha Cahill for volunteering her editing and proofreading skills. Thanks to Peg Mulqueen for reading the manuscript and giving me the green light and courage to move forward with publishing it. Thanks to Bridget Morris, Bella Forte Book Binding and Letterpress, for her exceptional talent. Thanks to all my yoga students who have been so open and receptive to my teachings over the years. Your love and support has enabled me to develop and mature in my ability to convey the teachings of yoga to the point where this book has become a reality.

I bow to Sri K. Pattabhi Jois and the authors of the sacred texts who have been the true inspiration behind this book. I salute anyone who takes the time to read and benefit from the teachings presented in *Vayu Siddhi*.

Enjoy,
Om Namah Shivaya!

David

Dedication

Bowing to the Void-Minded Yogis
Who Came Before

The writing of this book has been inspired by such sacred texts as *The Hatha Yoga Pradipika, The Shiva Samhita, The Gheranda Samhita,* and select Tantras and Upanishads. The aspiring yogi will find nectar in the language of hatha yoga used in these texts, nectar in the teachings that convey the highest reverence for the knowledge that is won from the study of asana and pranayama, the two favorite subjects of students of ashtanga yoga.

The unknown authors of these texts were independent and courageous "bad man"[1] inward explorers and risk takers who went against the societal grain to plumb the depths of their bodies and minds in the service of yoga. Through practice they forged into the unknown; they experienced new, creative ways of awakening and embodying their inherent spiritual essence. These boundary-pushing, shamanic yogis pioneered many beautiful, unusual, and potent practices, and they found ways of piercing through the ignorant blindness of the repetitive, compulsive, suffering, mad, chaotic, raging world of samsara.

Centered in breathing they practiced with passion, intensity,

---

1   See "Bad Man" pg 139

devotion, and surrender, piercing through even the most challenging obstacles, wrestling, breathing, and praying their way to self-realization. The fruits of their explorations are the basis for the new, progressive exploration of the asana and pranayama techniques that make up today's practice of ashtanga yoga. Sri K. Pattabhi Jois's lifetime study and teaching of asana and pranayama techniques are part of this marvelous lineage of hatha yoga.

This video series/book is a bowing to the yogis that have come before, especially to Sri K. Pattabhi Jois. And it is also an offering to the aspiring yogi, a invitation to you to perfect the art of breathing as part of becoming fluent in the language of hatha yoga. May you undertake a serious study of yoga and add to the fierce hatha yoga lineage. May you solitarily dive into the practices to find your greatest gift, your unique aesthetic spirit and style, and share your essential truths with all beings.

Centralizing Yourself in Breath

The decision to consistently and loyally attend to your breathing is the most important single decision that you will ever make to ensure success in yoga. Your breath is connected to everything important about you, from the plainly visible, most practical physiological aspects of you to your hidden, essential, secret sacred depths.

Breath sustains your physical life, helps feed your cells, and maintains the health of your tissues, brain, organs, and nervous system. And the elusive skill of knowing how you feel, of being able to give honest expression to the full range of your emotions, depends in part on you being awake to the rhythms of your breathing. Your ability to love, to feel empathy, to wholly involve yourself in the beauty and challenges of relationship requires you to breathe, sometimes with freedom and gusto and other times painfully, effortfully, or fearfully, as best as you can.

Realizing the depths of your psyche, the extent of your spiritual dimensions, depends on you undertaking a practice of doggedly following the organic ebb and flow rhythms of your breathing, its regular pattern of arising and passing away within your chest. Your breath carries the messages from the gods; you perceive your innermost profound dreams and visions by way of breath, and breath helps you access the templates that show you how to fulfill your unique destiny, your essential reason for being alive.

Championing your breath is the key to truly enjoying the fruits of your yoga practice, because it is through caring about your breathing that your tapas, the shining devotional heat that is the fruit of your stubborn dedication and your pointed, daily toil, will yield its important inner rewards. In using this video series/book and working with your breath, I hope you will turn to and trust your breath during times of celebration and challenge, that you will learn what it is to cultivate healthy breathing habits, and view breath as the key to unlocking the secrets to all yoga techniques.

In presenting this material I aim to transform your ideas about the role that your breath can play in your daily practice, to see how the consciousness that you develop through breath awareness leads you into the greater spiritual context of your life. I aim to set your imagination ablaze on the vital subject of breathing as your principal source of self knowledge.

In seeing your breath as your best ally, you'll enter into a more conscious, honest, and joyous relationship with yourself through breathing. Yoga practice is nothing except to know and embrace your breath's ever-changing movements and patterns, to listen to its many voices speak in many different feeling tones ranging from the softest of whispers to the most profound anguish-filled wailings.

Through listening to the subtle melodies of the breath's beckoning song, you empty yourself of unwanted thought, and in a flash, your seemingly isolated experience of existence can be transformed into a cosmic vision of the absolutely interconnected wholeness of everything, everywhere, at all times. True absorption in breath leads the small you to vanish, and what remains is an all-inclusive vision of you as Self, as everything, as the only, cosmic, uninterrupted, unified entirety.

"Yes free breathing you do! No stiff breathing."[1]

– Sri K. Pattabhi Jois

---

1 Sri K. Pattabhi Jois (Guruji) was known for saying these words while teaching

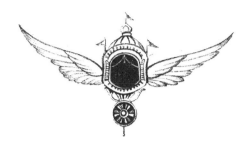

Getting Started

Three Steps to Learning Pranayama

This video series/book was born from two main themes:

(1) Ujjayi, the basic pranayama breathing, can be done by anyone at any time and under any circumstances. From *The Hatha Yoga Pradipika*: "Ujjayi breathing should be performed in all conditions of life, even while walking or sitting."[1] This indicates that there is no danger in lying down or sitting or otherwise studying the most natural thing you do, the act of breathing. And this is true regardless of your yoga experience level.

(2) It is almost miraculously helpful to think of the ashtanga practice as an equal combination of asana and pranayama. With the advent of his "breathing and movement system,"[2] Sri K. Pattabhi Jois boldly placed asana and pranayama together into one practice; he tapped the power of practicing the limbs together, and he put into practice that each limb shares a strong, proximate, and highly complementary relationship to the other. Limbs three and four, asana and pranayama, are two peas in a pod, two aspects of the same

---

1   *The Hatha Yoga Pradipika*   II-53
2   *Yoga Mala*   pg 37

practice, and by intentionally combining these two limbs
you can develop your practice with a welcome dynamism
and intensity that helps you burn through obstacles and
experience self-generated bliss.

Step One: Ujjayi Breathing
*(See video series, A Guide to Ujjayi Breathing, exercises 1 and
2, apana and prana. Also see "Ujjayi Breathing" on page 41 of
this book.)*

The first step to learning pranayama is to become highly
skilled at performing ujjayi breathing, to breathe with more
skill and awareness in your daily practice. Practicing with
the exercises in the ujjayi breathing video series will help you
to improve your ujjayi and gain more mastery of breathing
in practice. Even as a beginner you can work with the set of
introductory breathing exercises in this video series and use
your knowledge to develop your asana practice and better
prepare yourself for learning pranayama.

Step Two: Viloma Breathing
*(See video series, A Guide to Ujjayi Breathing, exercises 3–9 for
viloma breathing practice.)*

Viloma is the second most basic pranayama technique after
ujjayi and is a natural next step in the process of developing a
breathing practice. Viloma serves as a middle step between ujjayi,
the universal technique, and kumbhaka, the more advanced, main
pranayama technique. With viloma you further develop your
ujjayi breathing and at the same time you also make a small start in
kumbhaka. Each tiny interruption of the breath is a short retention
that can gradually help you to learn to suspend the breath.

Step Three: The Ashtanga Pranayama Sequence
(See video series, A Guide to the Pranayama Sequence.)

The sequence is presented in two sections: section one
provides detailed instruction on each of the five pranayamas in

the sequence; section two provides the uninterrupted ashtanga breathing sequence.

I suggest you learn the ashtanga breathing sequence by slowly working your way through the sequence in small increments, the same way that you learn the ashtanga asana sequences. For example you can begin by learning part A of the first pranayama called ujjayi:

Pranayama #1—Ujjayi: Parts A and B

To begin: *3 breaths*

Part A

(1) Exhale, control (retention)
(2) Inhale
Repeat steps 1 and 2 three times
(Transition to step 3 with no extra breaths)

(3) Inhale, control (retention)
(4) Exhale
Repeat steps 3 and 4 three times

3 breaths

Part B

(1) Inhale, control
(2) Exhale, control
Repeat steps 1 and 2 three times

3 breaths

At first your practice will be short, only two to four minutes long, but you can extend the time by repeating what you already know until you feel ready to move forward in the sequence. For example you can repeat part A, taking your time to thoroughly absorb it before moving on to part B. By patiently learning one portion at a time you will eventually learn the entire sequence. Your practice will become longer as you learn more, and the full sequence can take thirty to forty-five minutes or more to complete, depending on the length of your retentions.

When learning the different techniques of the five pranayamas, I suggest that you alternate between using the instructed portions and the uninterrupted portions of the video series, *A Guide to the Pranayama Sequence*. Use the instructed portion when you want to familiarize yourself with a pranayama technique such as bhastrika (pranayama #3) or when you want to receive extra instruction or tips on how to better approach the technique. Use the uninterrupted portion when you want to be guided through the sequence without interruption or extra instructions. You can turn off the video when you've reached your stopping place in the sequence, or you can repeat the sections that you've already learned.

Guidelines and Cautions

When practicing pranayama you can return to natural breath at any time. If you notice that your breathing feels forced, strained, out of control, or otherwise off, temporarily discontinue your work. Become receptive to your breath; allow it to come and go as it pleases and then restart your practice when you feel ready.

Return to natural breath:

(1) As the basic starting, returning, and ending point of your practice.

(2) When you've completed one or more sets of an exercise.

(3) When you find the exercise too difficult, or you get a sense that you can't keep up with the instruction.

(4) When your breathing becomes strained, or you feel fearful or a sense of panic, or like you are using excessive force.

(5) When you feel somehow overwhelmed, as though too much energy is being generated or built up. And when you feel excessive heat anywhere in the body but especially from the neck up.

(6) When you get fatigued or repeatedly lose focus.

(7) When you lose perspective or orientation on what you're doing.

(8) When you feel pressure or buzzing in the ears or head.

Extra guidelines for pranayama practice:

· The wise yogi works carefully, repeats the exercises, and trusts the process knowing that more ease will come with steady, diligent practice.

· The yogi breathes to look within, listen within, and feel within. He develops and fine-tunes his receptivity to the subtle breath, and he responds actively and positively to the momentary changes in the flow of his breathing and prana.

- The brain remains passive, the inner ears wide and receptive, the eyes calm, and the skin intelligent and soft.

- The steady-minded yogi adjusts her posture only when the need arises and only during rest intervals, otherwise she strikes an immovable spot and dives inward during pranayama practice. Patiently she seeks and finds the place where the breath flows deeply and spontaneously with the least effort.

The Power of Surrender and Receptivity

The void-minded yogi cultivates receptivity within the rigorous control aspect of her breathing practice by remembering that the Self, the wisdom within the body, is continually finding its way to express itself through her. And this happens independently of (at times in spite of) her sustained efforts to reach the Self.

The yogi receives breath as a gift; she enjoys its rhythmic sway that sweeps through her again and again.

She takes up practice each day with receptivity and ever-renews her opportunity to hear the breath's divine song calling to her from the depths within.

"For sixty years I have been forgetful, every minute,
but not for a second has this flowing toward me
stopped or slowed…."

— Rumi, "The Music"[41]

From an acceptance of her breath, she accepts an invitation to inner awareness. When this awareness becomes subtle enough she finds an invitation to observe the cosmic dance between purusa, pure consciousness, and prakriti, the active, agile dancer. The dancer takes center stage within the glorious axis, and the purity of her stainless dance is beheld by purusa, the Self in the ultimate act of communion. In order to be a witness to that rare, divine performance, the yogi empties her mind, empties her body, empties her breath, and bowing her head in reverent prostration, she receives the spectacular view of the sacred divine innermost dance of the Self.

---

1   *The Essential Rumi,* Translated by Coleman Barks

Sit Longer and With More Ease in Pranayama

One important part of pranayama is to establish and maintain a stable seat, or asana, and you can do this by orienting yourself along the vertical axis known as shushumna, most glorious. You will find a thorough exploration of this theme in the "Imagery for the Central Axis" section of this book (see page 25).

Sitting upright and focusing on your breath can create a surprising amount of tension throughout the body, particularly in the head, neck, and shoulder girdle. And so it is important to have strategies for relaxing and finding ease in your seated posture.

One strategy is to form a clear mental picture of your body's vertical alignment, imagining your head, torso, and pelvis as stacking up evenly along the central axis. Such imagery is done exclusively in the mind: You consciously refrain from using will or muscle power to achieve an upright posture, rather you work with images and allow the body to organize itself in accordance with the pictures you form through your posture. This can help you create an aligned position in a less effortful way, and you can tap your kinesthetic or more intuitive sense of how to maintain an upright posture for the duration of your breathing practice.

You can also improve your concentration, your posture, and thus your breathing by making periodic mental and visual scans of your head, neck, spine, hips, and legs in relation to the midline and to the earth. When you scan your posture pay particular attention to releasing the shoulders and neck or any other spot where you identify unnecessary tension. Periodically scanning and releasing any grip around the eyeballs or within the inner ears can help you cultivate a relaxed, receptive, or passive brain. Buzzing in the ears is a sign of strain and indicates a need to release tension.

Another such strategy for finding ease in your seated position is to start over by letting go of your conceptions of how to perform your posture. A return to home base or to a zero point, you figuratively shake down your body to release tension like shaking down a thermometer to reset it. This strategy can also be thought of as a return to emptiness, to a receptive state where you remember that you are simply sitting prayerfully, enjoying the rhythm of your breath, contemplating the silence in the gaps between breaths.

Additionally you can contemplate the classic image of the heart center, anahata, as a vast cave that expands outward in all directions, creating enough space within the torso to house the entire cosmos. This vast cave is eternally illuminated by the inexhaustible, unflickering, smokeless flame of the Self. Between breathing sets you can relax your effort and return to zero, to the vastness and restful sanctuary of the cave of the heart, releasing any residual tension, resetting your intention to make a fresh beginning. When you are ready, move your attention down the spine, start at your pelvic base, and work your way up the length of the spine through the mid torso, diaphragm area, to the shoulders, neck, and head.

Similarly in between each set of breathing exercises you can release jalandhara bandha (chin lock), relax your tongue and jaw in order to free your head, neck, and upper back. Then as you resettle into your position make sure that you align the palate and top of the sternum accurately over muladhara at the base. You can do this by imagining that the first rib circle between the collarbones lines up vertically over the pelvic floor.

When you are sitting in Padmasana it is advisable to change legs periodically or even frequently in order to refresh your seated position. If your legs become dull or begin to fall asleep, or if you experience any discomfort in your knees, then it is best to release your Padmasana, straighten the legs for a few moments, and retake your position with the opposite leg on top. Be patient and mindful of your body, slowly add to your pranayama sequence, and carefully cultivate your ability to sit for longer durations.

It is important to sit carefully and with awareness but also remember not to overcorrect yourself. It is possible to detract from your breathing and your practice by being overly critical of the small flaws in your seated position. At some point you must forget about creating the perfect seat, simply adopt your best posture, and allow yourself to be swept up into sacred ritual of following the great sound of the breath.

Setting Up a Seated Position

When setting up to sit for pranayama, nearly any upright position can be used. The material in the "Imagery for the Central Axis" section (see page 25) of the book provides a universal set of instructions that can be used for setting up any seated position for pranayama. Below I've included a few extra notes for sitting in Padmasana, Lotus posture, the best, most classic position for pranayama. These notes are a supplement to the video instruction on Padmasana in the *Vayu Siddhi* video series, *A Guide to the Pranayama Sequence*.

The following are instructions for sitting in Padmasana. These instructions will be given right leg first. However, in order to encourage balance and equal hip flexibility, I suggest you alternate legs (sometimes right leg first, sometimes left leg first). Change sides periodically during your pranayama practice particularly if your legs become tired, uneasy, or restless.

(1) Sit in Dandasana with a neutral pelvis that allows you to arrange your torso directly over the horizontal pelvic floor. Bend your right knee, close the knee joint as you bring the right heel up and in as close to the navel as you can get it.

(2) Keep the right heel up, into the navel, and direct your right knee forward to a 45 degree angle and down to the ground.

(3) Bend your left knee, close the knee joint, and place your left heel up and in as close to the navel as possible.

(4) Keep the left heel up and in and direct your left knee forward to 45 degrees and down toward the ground.

(5) Create an imaginary magnetic attraction between the knees, as though the knees are being drawn toward each other, and thus toward the midline.

(6) Imagine that your entire seated foundation (pelvis, thighs, shins, and feet) is magnetically attracted to the ground, stabilize your weight in your base, and physically lower your foundation toward the earth.

(7) Maintain your low, well-founded seat with the feet as high up the thighs as possible.

(8) Enjoy the containment of prana within your base, and appreciate the unequalled stability created by the legs being snugly crossed over each other. This unique leg mudra (seal, gesture) gives you a feeling of pelvic power, an internal grip within the center of your foundation.

(9) Keep the pelvic basin neutral by lifting the navel and lengthening the coccyx and see that you keep the sacrum into the body and vertical.

(10) Allow the spine to grow vertically out of the pelvis, circling upward like a lively creeper reaching for the sun.

(11) As you keep the navel up, also keep the front floating ribs down and into the body. Spread the wings of the kidneys and keep the back ribs wide.

(12) Lift up the chest from inside the torso. Feel that the lift is truly vertical, coming from within the torso along the spine. Align the manubrium (top of the sternum) over the xiphoid process (bottom of the sternum) over the pubic bone.

(13) Widen the collarbones, roll back the heads of the arms, and see that the shoulders remain evenly out to the sides of the body.

(14) Orient your shoulder position from the downward and inward action of the scapulae. Keep each scapula stamped into the body, feel them comfortably snugged into the body like two well-lodged, fitted base plates. Support the

expansion of the chest in front by attending to the scapular actions on the back side of the body.

(15) Balance your head vertically atop your neck and upper back. Relax the brain, broaden and empty the palate. Soften the eyes, maintain a downward gaze, and allow the inner ears to become spacious and receptive to the subtle sound of the breath. Maintain a clear connection between the root of the palate and the center of your well-founded seat. Enjoy an inner vastness, an utter bodily calm that is reflected in your relaxed facial demeanor.

Setting Up a Supine Position

For learning the exercises on *A guide to Ujjayi Breathing* of the video series/book, I recommend using a lying down position. A supine, lying down position enables you to passively open the chest and maintain the length of the spine and thus avoid the tension and fatigue that comes from the effort to sit up with spine erect. When you are first learning pranayama the lying down position can help you focus your energy more specifically on breathing.

Use a pranayama pillow or well-folded blanket to set yourself up so that you can press the feet into the wall with the legs straight. Lie back evenly on the support. Place a cushion or block under your head, making sure to adjust the height of the support with precision in order to achieve a distinct feeling of locking the chin in jalandhara bandha. Be careful to create just the right angle, not too much nor too little. This position ought to feel dynamic, like an open-chested lying-down Samastitihi position. Enjoy the ability to push the feet into the wall for added pelvic stability and thigh groundedness.

Also note that you want to set up your position so that you have a continuous downward slope from forehead to chin, chin to chest, chest to abdomen, abdomen to pelvic floor. This downward angle is important for relaxing the brain, getting the feeling for jalandhara bandha, and passively hollowing the belly in uddhyana bandha.

"Focusing the mind in a single direction is extremely important. To enable it to stay fixed and in place, Pranayama is essential."[1]

– Sri K. Pattabhi Jois

---

1   *Yoga Mala* pg 20

Imagery for the Central Axis

Optimizing Your Seated Position

You can use the imagery that I've provided in the following sections to better align yourself in any of the classic seated postures that are used for pranayama practice, including Padmasana, Virasana, Sukhasana or Baddhakonasana. Or you can use any other suitable alternative position that works for you, but remember to choose your pranayama seat carefully each time you practice. Be sure to adopt a position that enables you to sit tall with the head, torso, and hips in a true vertical line so that you can illuminate shushumna nadi through your study of breathing. The vertical axis can be thought of as spanning from the crown of the head down to the center of the pelvic floor and also upward from the pelvic floor to the crown. We'll start our imagery work at the base, the earth foundation.

The Pelvis

The pelvis is the foundation—home of muladhara chakra, location of mula bandha, and the cave of the sacrum. The foundation of your seat originates at the base of the spine within the lowest part of the pelvic basin at the location of the first chakra, muladhara (root support). The four corners of muladhara correspond to the four corners of the pelvic floor (1, pubic bone; 2, coccyx; 3 and 4, the two sitting bones) and are visually represented by a red four-petaled lotus flower. The number four is symbolic of stability, a strong foundation, and completeness, and thus the pelvic floor, with its four bony landmarks and the layers of muscle and connective tissue between them, form the basis of orientation for your pranayama seat.

Muladhara, the pelvic floor area, is also known as a yoni or womb. The yoni is a sacred feminine symbol of receptivity, and has several meanings including nest, receptacle, resting place, origin. Visualizing the pelvic floor as a yoni conveys the image of your lower center as a place of restful awareness, a sanctuary, a source of generative, creative energy, and of meditative retreat. Organize your head and torso vertically over muladhara.

Think of muladhara as your receptive, earth foundation. Align yourself as accurately as possible over or within the yoni, the sacred resting space delineated by the four boundary points of the pubic bone, coccyx, and two sitting bones. As you tune in to the base deep within the pelvis, also allow your awareness to extend outward to your legs in order to widen your base and thus broaden the feeling of your anchored seat. Increase your connection to the ground by feeling the legs as heavy, silent, and immovable. Imagine the legs and hips as set into or part of the ground as though they are an extension of it, an upwelling of earth emerging from below. Including the legs into the orientation of your foundation helps prevent unnecessary movement above in the torso, upper body, and head. As the legs and pelvis combine to tether you to the earth, feel your spine elongate and reach upward in response to this rooted, stable lower-body base.

The pelvic area is also known as the Apanastan, the home of apana vayu, out-breath pattern. The out-breath is said to culminate at a point or drop called bindu, located within the lower pelvis. This sacred point that culminates below the navel and above muladhara is said to be dimensionless, without a specific location, an esoteric link between the manifest world of mind, form, ideation, and the empty, transcendent void that is the abode of the Self beyond mind. The lower pelvis is known as the Apanastan because the seed or essence of the out-breath pattern is found there. By following the act of thoroughly emptying the lungs, the contraction of musculature helps you experience the condensation of energy into a single point within the pelvis. Experiment with this by emptying the lungs from the chest downward and see if you can refine your awareness by endeavoring to exhale down to a single point below the navel within the lower pelvis. Watch the downward and inward apanic energetic movement all the way to the end of the breath until you come to what can be thought of as a little seed, or an extracted essence of the out-breath pattern. There is a pure contractive quality in this essence, a very subtle, distinct, and powerful collection of energy within a tiny area of the pelvis. Then experiment with retaining the essence of the contractive, out-breath pattern as you initiate the in-breath. Carefully note the moment of finishing the exhalation and initiating the inhalation, and endeavor to retain the essence of the out-breath pattern as you begin to breathe in. Retain the seed of apana, hold to the kernel of residual contractive force as you begin to focus on the opposite pattern, the expansive, upward sweep of the inhalation. Notice the opposition between the two patterns; the apanic, contractive out-breath pattern and the pranic, expansive inhalation pattern. Remember to keep your awareness focused on a single point in the lower pelvis while you inhale as a means of helping to create a gentle suction that spans from the pelvic floor to the palate and helps to regulate the expansive sweep of the in-breath and to increase your lung capacity. Focusing on the centripetal, contractive qualities of the out-breath while breathing in is one way to activate mula bandha, the sealing-in of the apanic energy at your root or base.

The Sacrum

Another helpful key in working with the foundation of your seated posture is in coming to know the sacrum (literally the sacred bone). The sacrum is shaped like a downward-pointed arrow or a "V," and the tip of the V becomes the coccyx, or tailbone, that is actually a vestige of a very tiny tail. The sacrum joins the two halves of the pelvis in back, and it is important to orient your seat from this back portion of your pelvic foundation. The V stands for vertical because that's how you want to orient the sacrum in order to get a neutral pelvic base: the arrow points directly down and thus the pelvis remains level, neither tipping forward nor back. Finding a neutral base can be challenging because neutral might not feel like neutral, and so you can physically reach back to feel the sacrum as a means of getting an accurate feeling for neutral. You can experiment by exaggerating the tip of your pelvis forward back and then finding a neutral place between the exaggerations. This swinging forward and back of neutral can assist you in training your awareness to locate a more truly vertical aspect of the sacrum on the back side of the body.

You can also imagine that the arrow-shaped sacrum receives the transfer of weight from above, from the head down the spinal column to the base along the interior of the back side of the body. Imagine the interior of the back side of the body is inside the body, and notice the difference between this and imagining the back side of the body from the outside. Imagine that the added weight from above wedges the sacrum more snugly between the two halves of the pelvis (not unlike the keystone of a stone arch), increasing the stability of your seat as you sit. After transferring weight from above into the sacrum, the weight of the body continues downward into the two halves of the pelvis, and here the weight shifts slightly forward and then goes down vertically through the sitting bones and into the earth. You can imagine the pelvis as a basin or bowl, the two halves of the pelvis and the sacrum form the sides of the bowl and the pelvic floor forms the bottom of the bowl. Sit true and vertical for pranayama by imagining your pelvic basin as level all around, this includes the front, back, and sides. Imagine this stable, level basin as strong and powerful. This basin is easily able to support the weight of the head and spine above. Notice how freely and naturally the curved spinal column grows up plant-like out of this level basin, making it easy to keep the chest expanded and utilize the full capacity of your lungs.

In addition to its V shape the sacrum is also a thick bone, dished out from the inside forming a bony cave. This can help you to more clearly imagine the area of muladhara as a sacred, cave-like, spacious area. Imagining the cave-like shape of the sacrum can help you to experience the important circular energetic movement that you cultivate to initiate the inhalation. You can think of starting your inhalation by scooping or cleaning out this cave. Feel the beginning of each inhalation as a tiny, circular, upward swirl within the pelvis and you will understand uddhyana bandha. The action of energetically cleaning out the sacrum with the in-breath is also known as uddhyana bandha, a sucking back and up of the belly toward the spine.

The sacrum can also be thought of as one of the three sacred caves situated along the glorious axis: (1) the cave of the sacrum, (2) the cave of heart, and (3) the cave of the mouth.

Using this imagery, carefully balance your head and torso over your pelvic base, feeling the sacrum, the two halves of the pelvis, and the sitting bones as a wide base, an anchor that tethers you securely to the earth. See how aiming your awareness down the body into this base helps you experience your seat as an immovable spot, a spot of communion.

Mid Torso

The mid torso is the home of the diaphragm, manipura and anahata chakras, and the vast cave of the heart. After establishing your base, shift your focus up the central axis to the belly, kidneys, diaphragm, and rib cage. As you arrange your seat think of "relaxing the kidneys" and allow the back ribs to widen. Do this while using caution to confine this widening feeling to the mid torso and thus to maintain the level, neutral stability of your pelvic base. Relaxing and widening the kidneys is an instruction that contrasts and corrects what is known as collapsing the kidneys. This means to refrain from holding yourself rigidly upright by tensing the kidneys or overly pushing them up and forward into the body in an effort to open the chest. There is a middle spot between slouching and hypervigilance; the image of relaxing the kidneys back is more helpful if you tend to sit too far forward in a hypervigilant effort to open the chest. This can happen especially if you have a flexible spinal column. Awareness of widening and releasing the back side of the body can help you to hunker down, connect deeply with ground, and thus sit directly on the sitting bones instead of sitting perched too far forward. Relaxing the kidneys will not be as helpful if you already tend to sit too far back, and if you have trouble opening the chest as you sit. You want to find the middle place and stabilize your spine at the level of the mid torso. Learning to sense your kidneys in space can be of great assistance in arranging your torso along the vertical center line. You can correct your mid torso as you are sitting during practice by being receptive to the central axis, and working with the imagery of transferring the weight vertically down from the head to the tail, widening or energizing the kidneys, and releasing the front, lower, floating ribs downward. The ability to know if you are finding the middle between overly lifting and thus collapsing or overly widening and thus dropping the kidneys offers a fascinating, vexing, proprioceptive challenge that is partly based on long-held, preset ideas about what it means to sit up straight or to open your chest. At times it can be helpful to use a mirror, video, photographs, or a knowledgeable teacher to help you accurately align your position.

Focusing on the front side of the body can also offer another helpful image for aligning the middle portion of the torso; you relax the front floating ribs downward and this complements the back side image of relaxing and widening the kidneys. The image is to relax the front floating ribs downward toward the two frontal hip bones (anterior superior iliac spines—ASIS). You can palpate these two frontal hip bones by placing your index fingers on your navel and moving the hands apart from each other to the sides about three inches. Then move your fingers vertically down another inch or so to find each ASIS. You want to imagine that the two frontal hip bones have a secret message that they want to give to the floating ribs; picture them moving up toward the floating ribs in their effort to deliver this message. The floating ribs are intrigued and agreeable to receiving this message, and thus they remain pointed downward, lodged within the torso, at home, instead of lifting up and out as you attempt to open your chest. You can imagine a positive, magnetic attraction between the floating ribs and two frontal hip bones where the ribs are heavy and downward and the two pelvic bones circle upward in a gesture that complements the lift of the navel that is uddhyana bandha. Working with the image of the magnetic attraction between these two points has the effect of partly closing or shortening the abdomen area and will change the feeling of how to lift up your chest attempting to open it.

Another way to think about this area of the body is to think of the top rim of the pelvis and the bottom outlet of the rib cage as two flashlights. The pelvic rim flashlight shines vertically up and the bottom outlet of the ribs flashlight shines vertically down. The light from the two flashlights shine in a direct vertical line over each other. If you over lift your chest and eject the floating ribs up and out, your flashlights will no longer shine vertically over each other, and the floating rib flashlight will point down and back instead of vertical. Another way to think about it is not to allow the lower ribs to get caught up in what the upper sternum is doing. As you project the upper sternum forward and up, relax the front floating ribs down and in.

Also in this area you can visualize the horizontal aspect of the diaphragm, imagining it as a large horizontal sheet. Particularly emphasize this horizontal aspect as you work with the rhythm of the breath. During the inhalation watch the entire sheet move horizontally downward, and during exhalation, horizontally upward. With relative ease you can sense the extent of the diaphragm's sheet-like, horizontal width that spans the entire torso. Think of the diaphragm as aligning in a direct vertical line over its smaller brother the pelvic floor, and below the broad dome-like palate above. As you inhale, the diaphragm's broad horizontal surface area descends, widens, and flattens. You can enhance the feeling of the diaphragm's central positioning if you imagine that the back portions of the diaphragm widen and flatten more than the front when you inhale. With each breath there is a horizontal upward (exhalation) and downward (inhalation) excursion within the center of the torso. Think of the diaphragm's entire surface remaining parallel to the earth as a means of keeping the front floating ribs down and widening the kidneys back to facilitate alignment of the mid torso as you open your chest during pranayama.

This mid torso area is home of the third chakra, manipura (literally the city of jewels), the fire chakra. When you perform mula bandha at the base, you aim to seal your prana inward, and redirect it upwards. Then interiorized prana becomes a vital, illuminative inner force that lights up the solar plexus area like a city of jewels. The heat generated by skillfully redirecting prana to this area of the body increases the digestive fire and thus promotes internal cleansing and purification of the organs. Similarly, when you perform jalandhara bandha at the throat, you aim to redirect the upward energy of prana vayu downward. Successfully redirecting apana upward and prana downward helps you light up the city of jewels, causing this area to shine and bringing a sense of vitality and intelligence to the mid torso.

If you concentrate your attention a bit further up the central axis you come to the level of anahata, the heart center. Here you find the Pranastan, or home of prana vayu that exists in direct correspondence to the Apanastan that was described earlier. The esoteric Pranastan is where the seed, or the essence, of the in-breath pattern resides. Whereas apana is centripetal, contractive, inward, prana is centrifugal, expansive, outward. One practice is to keep your attention fixed in the Pranastan, in the essence of the expansive pattern whose home is in the heart center during the out-breath. This means that you retain the essence of prana vayu, of the upward, outward in-breath pattern as you exhale, and you do this by continuing to lift up and expand the chest while breathing out. To retain the essence of the pranic inhalation during the exhalation you focus your attention in the heart center and keep the chest open as you empty the lungs. Notice that the lift of the chest during exhalation balances the downward and inward squeeze of apana vayu. Keeping the chest expanded by retaining the essence of the in-breath pattern counters the downward and inward squeeze of the out-breath pattern. Remaining within the Pranastan reduces the undesirable tendency for the chest to deflate and collapse during exhalation.

The imagery pertaining to maintaining awareness of the opposite vayu pattern during breathing forms a major theme in attaining vayu siddhi, mastery of the vayu patterns of breathing. There is a refinement of awareness that takes place in gaining knowledge of the opposing play of vayus by studying the rhythmic, cyclic patterns of the breath. The first two exercises of the video series, *A Guide to Ujjayi Breathing* focus on understanding the movement patterns of apana and prana vayus.

Within the heart center you find the grand image of the cave of the heart that is eloquently and poetically described in the sacred texts. The heart's cave is described as a vast, dimensionless inner realm, a sacred cave that contains the Void, vast space. The cave of the heart contains all of existence, including the eternal, endless cycles of creation, preservation, and dissolution. Amidst the ceaseless, cyclical activity of nature, prakriti, you can find the Self dwelling in the central cave of heart. It is thought of as the size of a thumb. The atman dwells in the cave of the heart; it is known as the ineffable, secret one, the individualized, in-dwelling Self, and it is symbolized as residing in the cave of the heart in the form of a smokeless, unflickering flame that never burns down. This eternal light illuminates the entire inner world with its brilliant, unfaltering light of compassion and intelligence.

Upper Body

The upper body comprises the top of the chest, neck, and head, and vishuddhi and ajna chakras. Moving up from the mid torso you come to the first rib circle, vocal folds, neck, palate, root of the palate, and head. The throat area is a key area for breathing. The sound of ujjayi breathing is produced by partially closing the glottis, a narrowing of the space between the vocal folds. You want to work to become skilled in manipulating the throat to create a dynamic, fluid, resonant, and inviting sound that helps you interiorize your awareness of breath's ever-repeating cycle. Part of using the breath to concentrate the mind is using the breath's sound to transfer your attention from outside to inside the body through interior listening—opening the inner ears and withdrawing the mind into the middle channel, the subtle aspect of the spinal column.

Creating resistance in the throat helps you learn to regulate the breath, to control the speed and volume of the in- and out-breaths. You can use this control of the breath to internalize your awareness along the central axis by causing the breath to travel up and down along the middle channel from the base to the root of the palate with slow, steady, expansive inhalations, and even, long, contractive exhalations. The throat area is also key for learning to vertically align the head, neck, shoulders, and upper torso directly over the lower spine and pelvis. The glottis is located near the first rib circle, where the rib cage begins at the top of the chest, and both the first rib circle and the vocal folds can be imagined as horizontal surfaces that you endeavor to align directly over the center of the diaphragm, the bowl of the pelvis, and the pelvic floor. Utilizing this imagery can give you excellent results in creating postural awareness in an area of the body that requires perceptive subtle awareness in order to create and sustain alignment. The throat is where vishuddhi (purity) chakra is located. You can imagine the ascending vertical arrangement of chakras from muladhara at the base, to manipura above the navel, to anahata at the heart center, up through the throat area at vishuddhi as a means of creating clear postural and meditative alignment along the middle line.

Moving up you come to the third sacred cave, the cave of the mouth. The broad palate area that forms the roof of the mouth is part of an entire esoteric area known as Khecari. The suction of the in-breath that is a result of narrowing the glottis helps you feel the entire mouth as a broad, deep, dome-shaped mountain yoga cave, like Shiva's abode or a vaulted ceiling in a great stone cathedral. During inhalation the back of the throat fans open and broadens as when you yawn, and the palate is activated as when sipping in the nectar-like sweetness of a thick beverage, such as a milkshake. Breathing in from the base by using the suction of the in-breath to empty the palate helps you cultivate a discerning palate, a fine inward awareness, a more subtle appreciation of the alignment principles that help you to organize your head over your torso and pelvis.

The area above the palate, in the sinus's behind the bridge of the nose is also known as khecari, or the root of the palate. The exact location of khecari can be thought of as elusive, esoteric, imaginative, or variable. Sometimes khecari is simply the spacious roof of the mouth and sometimes you can experience it as more confined to a more subtle, smaller upper area known as the root of the palate. This area corresponds with ajna, the sixth chakra, the command center. It is thought of as the upper terminus of shushumna, the mountain axis that begins at muladhara at the base. Proper vertical alignment is facilitated by imagining a direct, uninterrupted, two-direction (from down to up and from up to down) line of communication between muladhara at the base and the root of palate, khecari, at the peak. Imagine that the root of the palate and the pelvic root support, which are at opposite ends of the same pole, engage in an ongoing dialogue; they communicate with each other directly, like an express line without an intermediary. The two ends of the poles work closely together to ensure that the integrity of the vertical line is maintained as you sit and go inward to focus on your breathing. (See also "Khecari Mudra" on page 76 of this book.)

Sahasra is a major image, a significant piece of puzzle in the inner mapping of shushumna that helps the yogi transform the body into a divine temple within. Using sahasra, the yogi envisions the entire span of shushumna and creates an inner sacrificial fire along this world axis. Here the flame of continuous awareness that is meditation burns and gives the inner view, the inner seeing that becomes a wide and round view—a soulful, wise, and compassionate consciousness, as opposed to a right, pointed, linear, and narrow consciousness.

The upward movement of illuminated Shakti, free from the fetters of ego and whose light is as brilliant as a million moons, begins at the base and culminates at this highest point. This goddess, symbolizing the emergence of the highest, self-reflective inner attunement, is no longer sleeping nor hindered and hidden down in the depths. Now she stands up along the central axis and enjoys the view from her central, sacred place with consciousness.

This is the image used by the yogi for optimally orienting and aligning the body along the central axis in asana and pranayama practice. Clarifying the line from muladhara to sahasra helps the yogi to strike that single sacred stance that stuns or paralyzes the hindering, conflicting inner forces long enough to receive glimpses of that ever-renewing spectacular view. The base of shushumna is kundalini's initial sleeping and starting place; the top of the world mountain, shushumna is Shiva's divine seat. Through awakening, containing, and raising up his life energy, the yogi aims at reuniting the goddess power with Shiva, the auspicious, at sahasra, thus bringing about the new beginning where receptivity reigns and an appreciation of the power and significance of the inner world brings forth an enlightened state overflowing with nectar.

"...the breath brought under control, little by little, by the strength of one's practice, difficult though this is, it is possible."[1]

– Sri K. Pattabhi Jois

Ujjayi Breathing

The diaphragm is the main muscle involved in breathing; when you can get an experiential feeling of its actions, that knowledge helps you breathe better.

You can learn to sense the diaphragm's anatomical location within the torso and to follow its contraction (inhalation) and relaxation (exhalation) phases. The diaphragm is a large sheet or dome-shaped muscle that resembles a mushroom or a parachute, and divides the upper and lower abdomen. It has an unattached gathering of fibers called the central tendon at its top that helps give it its dome shape. It attaches to several sets of ribs and has two stems called crura that attach to vertebrae along the front of the lower spine. The diaphragm is both a particularly large muscle and a core muscle. This is significant because it means that its rhythm and its actions and movements are quite easy to observe. And this basic observation serves as a vehicle that takes you into the root and center of you.

Here's an image for you to work with: your torso is a vast inner ocean. Imagine that the diaphragm is a giant jelly fish that is entirely at home floating up and down on the ocean currents within your torso. As you inhale its fibers contract and move down, flatten and spread, and as you exhale its fibers relax, move up, bunch together, and re-form their dome-like shape. Allow your mind to enjoy the steady, easy, rhythmic movement of this large sheet-like muscle, and tune into its actions again and again within your torso.

The piston-like repetitive rhythm of the diaphragm within your torso's center can help you in discovering mula bandha. The expansion and contraction of the diaphragm can show you the workings of the pelvic floor. The pelvic floor moves in rhythm with the actions of the diaphragm. Both the pelvic floor and the diaphragm are horizontal, sheet-like surfaces within the torso, one large (diaphragm) and one small (the pelvic floor). These two areas share a synergy. They act symphonically; tuning into the larger, grosser one helps you tune in to the smaller, subtler one.

An elusive, esoteric, and challenging practice such as mula bandha can be accessed with more ease and more logic when you approach it through observing the diaphragm. As you watch the rise and fall, expansion and contraction, you can better understand how to effectively seal the pelvic floor in order to pull up and redirect apana vayu. Mula bandha is often defined as forcibly pulling up apana vayu, and causing the otherwise downward apanic energy to flow upward. The upward movement of the diaphragm during exhalation provides you with the means of finding the redirection, the against the grain energetic upward direction of mula bandha.

You can pull up apana and achieve mula bandha by causing your perineum to ride on the coattails of the diaphragm as it ascends the torso when you exhale thoroughly. Following these rhythms is what trains you to master your senses by remaining present in the center in order to listen, feel, and see within in a sustained manner.

The diaphragm is a major ally in an often long and slow process of winning the ability to withdraw your senses and sustain your attention along the central axis. When you observe the vertical action of the diaphragm and its influence on the pelvic floor, you can align yourself more easily along the central axis known as the pillar of light, or shushumna nadi. To be able to sustain your focus along the center line of the body from the base through the crown is one of the purposes for practicing pranayama.

The type of authentic breath that can take you into meditation can be accessed simply by observing the diaphragm within your torso and understanding how to optimize its muscular actions. You'll also eventually see how to shape and guide the movements of this large muscle, and how that skill leads to awareness of the more subtle physical actions such as the relationship between breathing patterns and awakening the pelvic floor (mula bandha).

And there's more—because the diaphragm drives the ever-repeating cycle of the breath, it has a major role in helping you understand vinyasa. When you study the diaphragm you study vinyasa from a central vantage point; through breathing you follow the opposing movement patterns that make up the ashtanga sequences. In ashtanga yoga practice, through combining vinyasa and breathing, you endeavor to generate and to harness the dynamic biorhythms at the heart of you. That is why Sri K. Pattabhi Jois called ashtanga a breathing and movement system. The most accessible way to get to the heart of the rhythm of this breathing and movement system is to doggedly follow the actions of the diaphragm and see how those actions translate into vinyasa, into rhythmic opposing movement patterns.

See if you can follow the diaphragm's piston-like, vertical up-and-down action within the torso as you focus on the connection between rhythm in breathing and rhythm in creating actions in your asanas and in your movement transitions. Each time you effectively tune into the true, deep rhythm of your breath, you are in position to have some small epiphany about your movement and posture at its source. You can get some small flash of surprise—perhaps an insight into how to move more like you, with more spirit and intelligence.

Nine Keys to
Better Ujjayi Breathing

(1) Ujjayi sound breathing is done by partially closing the glottis—the space between the vocal folds—as when you swallow, whisper, or yawn.

(2) Follow the sound of your exhalation by whispering the syllable ham; draw out the syllable, make it long: "Haaaaaaaammmmmm." You can do it with the mouth open or closed. Repeat until you feel comfortable simultaneously narrowing your throat, contracting your abdomen, and producing a long hissing sound to empty your lungs.

(3) Breathe in by imagining that you have no nose or mouth and pretend to draw the breath in through a hole in the throat. Use this method to broaden the palate and feel the pull of the breath across the throat.

(4) The out-breath is a gentle squeeze that you can feel as a friendly push from the top of chest, down through the narrowing rib cage, into the withdrawing abdomen, and inward to the base of the pelvis. Refine the squeeze so that it matches the even, rhythmic flow of the breath. Synchronize the smooth sound of your exhalation with the steady contractile squeeze of your ribs and abdomen.

(5) The in-breath can be experienced as a powerful pull activated by narrowing the throat and cultivating a gentle suction. This results in a circling of the inhalation behind the navel and up to the widening kidneys, into the broadening ribs, and finally expanding the chest to mighty capacity.

(6) The diaphragm moves up and down along the vertical central axis within the center of your torso with piston-like regularity. During the inhalation watch your dome-shaped diaphragm contract, flatten, widen, and move down the torso. And during the exhalation observe the diaphragm

release, narrow, move up and assume its original dome-like shape. Use your awareness of the diaphragm's movements within the torso to regulate your breath, to skillfully synchronize the sound with the speed of the breath.

(7) Align the sound of your ujjayi breathing with the directional movements of prana and apana vayus. Listen and follow the apanic route of the out-breath as it sweeps down the spine and into the yoni at the pelvic floor base. Follow the route of the pranic in-breath by following it up and behind the belly; listen to the upward sweep of the expansive in-breath to the top of the chest.

(8) To renew the sound of your breath, relax the brain, soften the eyes, and release the eyelids. Cultivate receptivity within the inner ears. Touch the middle portion of the tongue to the roof of the mouth, broaden the palate, release the root of the tongue, soften the jaw, and sip the nectar of breath.

(9) Finally, simultaneously watch and listen to the ever-renewing cycle of glorious rhythmic breathing within you. Tune into the twin sounds of the inseparable pair of opposites whose powerful energetic presence and central location within the torso provide the single most potent means of gaining inward-directed consciousness.

Prana and Apana Vayus:
The Highest Agents

In *The Yoga Sutras* the pairs of opposites are known as dvandas, and asana work leads the well-grounded yogi to stay rooted in his stance in the face of any sort of contradictory forces that manifest within him. Asana mastery requires the yogi to maximize his understanding of opposing forces, and he accomplishes this initially by clarifying and defining each separate force. The ability to clearly distinguish each pole of an opposing force is what eventually leads the yogi to create subtle, meditative awareness. He appreciates the nuance and finesse that creates the subtle dynamism of playing one force against another. This discernment leads him to a new stance, an unbiased center position between the pairs of opposing actions.

Prana and apana are the classic pair of opposites. Shiva calls them the highest agents because they provide the most central, direct, and accessible means of understanding how to work with opposition in yoga practice. Thus, the approach that the wise yogi takes in working with the two highest agents becomes the prototype for working with all forms of opposition within himself: physical, emotional, analytical, reflective, and finally spiritual.

Apana Vayu

Apana vayu governs the lower abdominal and pelvic region within the torso from the navel to the pelvic floor. Linked with the out-breath, the apanic pattern is a downward, inward, cohesive, centripetal force that has rooting and grounding propensities. The force of apana is a predominant natural force that is evident in the downward growth of plants, in the root systems that live in earth, provide nourishment, and serve to support and tether the plant securely to the ground. This force is also evident in the descent of a child from the womb, the digestive elimination, and the powerful downward course of a water fall.

By tuning into the pattern of apana vayu, the investigative yogi gains full knowledge of the intricacies of exhaling, including utilizing the full extent of subtle breathing muscles within the abdomen, pelvis, and pelvic floor. Understanding apana vayu, the movement pattern of the exhalation, helps the sadhaka to cleanse and purify the network of nadis, pranic channels that snake throughout the body. Working with apana during pranayama practice helps the yogi to gain a reverence for the earth, to experience the ground as generous and trustworthy, an inexhaustible source of abundance. Stopping the downward course of apana vayu and redirecting it upward toward samana vayu in the belly is mula bandha.

Prana Vayu

Prana vayu governs the region of the chest cavity from the diaphragm to the collarbones and includes the lungs, rib cage, and entire upper torso. Linked with the in-breath, the pranic pattern is an upward, expansive, centrifugal, opening pattern. The force of prana vayu is evident in the blossoming and flowering of plants and in their expansive reach upward toward sunlight; in the flight of a bird away from the earth; in the rise of a fast moving arcing ocean wave; and in the whirling funnel of a cyclone. Working with the pranic pattern during inhalation helps you elongate along the central axis and encourages spaciousness and receptivity within the torso. Stopping the upward course of prana vayu and redirecting it downward into the belly (samana vayu) is called jalandhara bandha.

The skillful yogi learns to recognize the upward expansive prana vayu pattern and thus gains mastery over the intake of prana into her body. She learns to draw the breath in with precision and subtle suction along the middle axis. Similarly she understands and directs the downward course of apana vayu by cultivating a slow, steady hissing sound when exhaling. Knowledge of the course of the exhalation from the heart center down to the base of the pelvis causes the mind to withdraw inward to the central axis. Through work with the two highest agents, breath control (pranayama) becomes vayu control (vayu siddhi), and vayu control becomes mind control (samadhi).

Sri K. Pattabhi Jois (Guruji) said "becoming skilled in pranayama enables one to take in the subtle power of the vital wind."[1] This refers to controlling prana and apana vayus. Through pranayama the aspirant is able to tap and control the power contained in the interiorized prana called vayu, or vital wind.

In order to take subtle control of the power of the vital wind, the yogi unwaveringly observes his breath's play; he awakens

---

1   *Yoga Mala* pg 23

his mind to the breath's rhythmic swing from pranic pole to apanic pole. He regulates this grand rhythm and causes the activities of his mind to align with his breathing. As the breath becomes steady so too does the mind, and both become free from disruption, interference, or disturbance.

Through the medium of dynamic breathing the yogi harnesses the opposing forces within himself, plays with the infinite pairs of opposites, learns to create dynamism in asana and pranayama by causing one force to act against its opposite in an unceasing dance that is both subtle and intelligent. The purpose of practice is for the fortunate yogi to direct the vayu poles of the breath and routinely experience full-body pranic awakenings that transform his inner energy.

Prana and Apana Vayu Exercises

I suggest you take time to get to know the vayu patterns of prana and apana separately. You can do this by working with the first two exercises in the video series, *A Guide to Ujjayi Breathing*. After you get a good feeling for each of these patterns, I then invite you to turn your attention to a further, more subtle application of the vayu patterns to breathing, and that is to begin to observe the interdependent relationship between the two patterns. Instead of perceiving each pattern, each half of the breath as a separate event, you begin to observe the two patterns as an interaction between opposing forces. This is where the concept of bandhas interfaces with breathing, as when you create mula bandha by exhaling thoroughly and redirecting the downward course of apana vayu upward and jalandhara bandha by inhaling thoroughly and redirecting the upward course of prana vayu downward.

It is important to note that when working with breathing and with bandhas you should orient yourself vertically in relationship to the earth. It is important to emphasize the vertical upward and downward directions of breathing and the corresponding opposite direction of the bandhas. For understanding the bandhas it is helpful to perceive upward movement within downward movement, and downward movement within upward movement. Understanding the bandhas will come to you much more easily if you simply think of the fundamental directions (up and down) as happening at the same time and as opposing each other.

Below you will find two excerpts taken from exercises one and two in the video series, *A Guide to Ujjayi Breathing*. These written notes are meant to give you an alternate means of absorbing the information on the fundamental theme of identifying the patterns of breathing while attending to the opposing directions of the bandhas. After reading and studying these notes I suggest you practice again along with the video and see if you are able to further define and clarify your understanding of the vayu patterns and the oppositional relationship that creates bandhas.

Breathing actions that redirect apana upward.

Turn your attention to the upward actions that contrast the downward apanic movement of exhaling. Get ready by inhaling deeply and prepare to work with the out-breath:

- Exhale; activate the feet and legs, lift the foot arches and kneecaps. Ground and firm the thighs. Feel energy move up the legs as though to support the pelvis as you thoroughly empty the lungs to your base.
  Inhale... and try again.

- Exhale; from the peak downward and lift the root at the pelvic floor feel as if you are pulling up apana, redirecting its downward flow upward.
  Inhale... and try again.

- Exhale; focus on closing the root at muladhara and containing the energy of the out-breath, apana, within the pelvis...
  Inhale from this base to the top of the chest and try again.

- Exhale; stay in contact with the ascent of the diaphragm. Allow its upward movement to float the center of the perineum up against the downward flow of exhaling.
  Inhale evenly.

- Exhale; seal muladhara, pull up apana, lift the navel and sternum, redirect the energy upward...
  Inhale, smooth and steady... and try again.

- Exhale; with jalandhara bandha plant the legs, perform mula bandha, redirect the energy at the root, and lift the chest...
  Inhale.

- Exhale; keep the brain passive and feel the two opposite directions of action along the middle axis.

Here's a review of the upward actions:

- Lift the arches of the feet away from the wall (if in supine position).

- Lift the knee caps and thigh muscles (if in supine position).

- Lift up muladhara, the center of the pelvic floor. Feel as if you are stopping the descending, apanic energy of the out-breath and thus creating rooted, dynamic support at your base.

- Lift the navel back toward the spine and upward away from the pubic bone to create uddhyana bandha.

- Observe the upward movement of the diaphragm during exhalation and imagine that the center of the perineum is attached to the diaphragm by a thin thread and thus follows the diaphragm upward into the body.

- Float the heart upward and expand the chest as you watch the descending, inward direction of the out-breath.

Actions that oppose prana vayu:

- Turn your attention to the downward actions along the body that contrast the upward pranic movement of inhaling.

- Breathe in and feel the forehead, skin of the face, eyes, and chin sloping downward; feel this in contrast to the upward expansion of the in-breath. These actions create jalandhara bandha, or chin lock, to counter the rising energy of the in-breath.
  Exhale evenly along the central axis to the pelvic floor and try again.

- Observe the in-breath from the perspective of the downward slope of the face and head. Lowering the forehead and chin helps you redirect the upward energy of inhalation downward, and this action contains prana within the torso rather than allowing it to escape up and out as you breathe in.
  Exhale smoothly down to your base.

- As you draw a breath in from the lower pelvis watch your coccyx lengthen, descend, and curl inward toward the pelvic floor. Feel this action in contrast to the strong upward movement of the in-breath and the belly.
  Exhale.

- Draw the breath in circularly, follow the route up the back side of the body, and use the breath to spread the wings of the kidneys.
  We'll do two more breaths, exhale.

- As you breathe in feel the upward direction of the in-breath contrasted by the downward pressure of the feet into the wall (if in supine position). Lengthen your tail as you lift the navel, widen the back ribs, lower the eyes, and feel the downward slope of the forehead. Become absorbed in the play of contrasting directions.
  Exhale long and slow, hollowing the belly.

- Breathe in lifting the foot arches (if in supine position), kneecaps, perineum, navel, and sternum; feel the weight and length of your tail as you redirect the strong flow of upward energy downward with jalandhara bandha.

- Feel the increased ability to center yourself, to inhabit your body, as you become skilled at perceiving the opposing actions and counteractions within the vayu patterns that arise with the cycle of the breath.

"Through the practice of Pranayama the mind becomes trained in a single direction and follows the movements of the breath."[1]

– Sri K. Pattabhi Jois

---

1   *Yoga Mala* pg 23

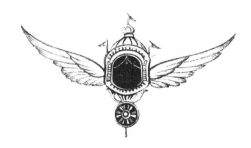

Mudras

Uddhyana Bandha Kriya

Uddhyana: to fly up (referring to sucking up of the abdomen).
Bandha: lift, close, redirect.
Kriya: cleansing action, purifying practice.

Uddhyana bandha kriya is one of six kriyas, or cleansing actions, that are commonly performed in classical hatha yoga. The technique consists of flushing the air out of your lungs, suspending your breath, and pulling up your entire abdomen so that your belly flies up, and becomes hollow. You hold the breath and attempt to touch the navel to the spine. This kriya can be practiced with relative ease by beginners, and so it often serves as an unofficial introduction to kumbhaka (retention).

The importance of uddhyana bandha kriya as a teacher of breathing, bandhas, and core activation cannot be overstated. It might be the most potent, significant single yoga technique, and practicing it can help you with the following:

(1) Learn to breathe out more thoroughly, thus to reclaim the power of your breath, to breathe more as you are meant to breathe.

(2) Engage your belly and pelvic muscles more intentionally and thoroughly.

(3) Become more dynamic, animal-like, graceful, and emotionally expressive in your movements and postures.

(4) Better understand how to seal in your prana, life force, at the base, and thus redirect apana vayu upward (mula bandha).

(5) Have a powerful, active, intelligent center that helps you skillfully apply the essential hatha yoga techniques for mind control and well-being.

(6) Lift your navel and lower abdomen as a main way of awakening muladhara (the root support chakra) within the pelvis, and thus illuminating the central axis from the base upward.

(7) Experience your center as a wellspring source of dynamic power for awakening buddhi (fine, discerning intellect) and entering into more subtle states of meditative awareness.

(8) Learn to pull up the perineal body, and thus perform the subtle actions of mula bandha.

(9) Have better digestion, prevent sickness and disease; have more beautiful skin and a more slender waist.

(10) Attain vayu siddhi, mastery of the movements of prana within your body; win more capacity to direct your energy, better choose your reactions to emotions and thoughts; connect steadying your breath with steadying your mind.

(11) Promote longevity.

(12) Train your awareness to repeatedly withdraw into shushumna, the glorious middle axis. Practicing uddhyana particularly helps you access the elusive base of the central axis.

(13) Have easy access to hatha yoga's most powerful secret techniques even if you are a beginner.

(14) Achieve the grayhound dog shape of the abdomen, a sacred shape that constitutes a powerful body yantra, a visual instrument, whose contemplation will help you establish a more profound connection between your physical expression and the subtle concentration of your mind in your asana work.

(15) Successfully adopt the uddhyana shape, and thus more thoroughly utilize your core to strike a stance that is a great energetic seal: a maha mudra, an earth-connected, immovable spot that brings steady breath, an empty palate, and a clear, pure mind.

(16) Refine the alignment of your asana positions through breathing as means of activating and toning the central, deeper, more powerful and influential core muscles.

(17) Transform your center into a source of great energetic vitality in practice by cultivating the dynamic use of your abdominal and pelvic breathing musculature, and thus develop the skill of breathing out.

Uddhyana Bandha Kriya
Set-Up Positions and Exercises

Position One

- Stand with your feet parallel and separated slightly wider than hip width.

- Bend the knees, sit down and back, and adopt a powerful stance like a skier going downhill.

- Place your hands on your thighs near the knees and keep the arms straight.

- Keep your head, eyes, and chin down throughout the exercise.

- Keep the chest gently open, flex the lumbar spine, and tip the pelvis slightly back (an action like a dog hiding his tail).

- Plant the feet and make a ready stance.

- When performing the kriya, push the hands down strongly onto the thighs keeping the arms straight—use the pressure between the arms and legs to get leverage to suck the abdomen back and up.

Position Two

Full Lotus (or equivalent: Half Lotus, crossed legged, supported on a cushion, Baddha Konasana, or Virasana)

Exercise One

- Take your set-up stance and get ready.

- Swiftly flush the air out of your lungs and don't breathe in.

- Push down on your thighs with your hands and keep the arms straight.

- Suck the entire belly back and up and remain in that position for as long as possible without straining.

- Keep the eyes and chin down. Look down at your abdomen to help get the feeling of making the belly area hollow.

- Let the lock go and release the belly before attempting to breathe in.

Get ready, and try again.

Empty the lungs with gusto and pause. Suck the entire abdomen up and again pause. Become absorbed inward as you stop the cycle of the breath. Explore the lift for as long as is possible without forcing. Release the lock and then slowly, smoothly breathe in. Maintain your form in between repetitions.

- Keep the eyes down, the knees bent, and the hips down and back.

Prepare, and try once more.

Swiftly empty the lungs and don't breathe in. Suck the belly upward by pushing down firmly on your thighs with straight arms. Enjoy the lift and the interval of suspended breath as long as is desired. Then release the lock and breathe in smooth and slow.

Carefully watch several breaths immediately following the set of locks. Let the sound of the breath be deep and smooth as you fill and empty the lungs slowly and completely. Feel the power and pervasive quality of the breath. And see if you can get more in touch with the patterns of prana and apana vayus as you breathe in and out respectively.

References from The Hatha Yoga Pradipika

- Uddhyana is so called by the yogis because by its practice the prana (vayu) flies (flows) in the shushumna.[1]

- Uddhyana is so called because the great bird prana, tied to it, flies without being fatigued.[2]

- The belly above the navel is pressed backward toward the spine. This uddhyana bandha is like a lion for the elephant of death.[3]

---

1 *The Hatha Yoga Pradipika* III–54
2 *The Hatha Yoga Pradipika* III–55
3 *The Hatha Yoga Pradipika* III–56

- Uddhyana is always very, very easy when learned from a Guru.[1]

- Of all the bandhas, uddhyana is the best; by binding it firmly liberation comes spontaneously.[2]

References from The Shiva Samhita
- Through practice of uddhyana bandha, vigraha siddhi (power over the microcosm) is obtained. Vayus are purified.[3]

1   *The Hatha Yoga Pradipika* III–57
2   *The Hatha Yoga Pradipika* III–59
3   *The Yoga Samhita* IV–51

Jalandhara Bandha

Jalandhara: net, support.

Bandha: lock, close, shut, redirect.

Chin Lock: net-holding lock. Like a fisherman would use to hold one end of his net beneath his chin, while casting out the rest of it.

Jalandhara bandha, the chin lock, is an essential ashtanga yoga technique. It is the upper most bandha of the three main bandhas. Its sphere of activity is in the region of the head, brain, palate, neck, and throat center along the middle axis of the body. By applying jalandhara bandha, you endeavor to stop the upward movement of prana vayu, the inhalation pattern, and also to redirect its expansive energy downward. Jalandhara bandha is a both a physical and energetic practice, and each of these aspects has its challenges and rewards.

The physical chin lock is performed by lifting the chest and lowering the chin firmly onto the notch between the collarbones. This seemingly straightforward action is actually quite challenging for many people, and thus success might require considerable contemplation and practice (see the "Jalandhara Bandha Gesture" section on page 66 for alternatives and modifications of the chin lock). The challenging part of performing jalandhara is to impressively expand the chest while maintaining the integrity of your seated posture and then to lower the chin far enough down to clamp onto the sternum without dropping the head too far forward and down. The action through the head, neck, and upper spine that creates jalandhara requires upper body flexibility, especially in the neck and jaw, and thus must be approached cautiously, patiently, and with a kinesthetic intelligence that enables you to maintain the proper alignment of your head in relation to your neck and upper spine. The reward of skillfully applying the chin lock is to win the ability to maintain a tall, energetically alive seat during pranayama, to acquire a discerning palate, and to position yourself for a spectacular view of the inhalation.

The energetic aspect. In order to become fluent in the energetic language of hatha yoga, you must repeatedly contemplate the role of jalandhara bandha as a stoppage of energy, a lock, a sealing in, and a redirection of energy. In containing life force within your torso from above you cause the prana inside the body to flow more freely through the nadis, the energetic circuitry of the body, and this becomes an ability to direct prana internally. Undirected prana escapes the body or becomes stuck or dormant or otherwise unavailable. The role of the three bandhas in pranayama is to prevent the escape of prana from the torso, to help awaken dormant, inactive prana, and to facilitate the directional flow of prana into wanted channels such as shushumna. Given its close proximity to the brain, the chin lock partly serves to activate the concentrative, inward-turning capacity of the mind. With jalandhara, by lowering the forehead, eyes, nose, jaw, and chin, you are creating an inward-turning gesture, a bowing down, an invitation to the brain to give up its nonessential incessant activity and instead become passive, observant, and receptive, absorbed in the patterns of thought that lead toward a cessation of thought.

Below you will find a set of written instructions for attaining success in this challenging mudra.

Begin at the base. Arrange your seat from the earth and then proceed up the spine. Start at the pelvic floor; make sure you have a stable neutral base by sitting directly on the sitting bones. Feel the vertical axis of the body. Your jalandhara bandha will be compromised if you are sitting with the pelvis tilted backward or forward.

Tips for expanding the chest. As you lift and broaden the chest also widen the mid back. Expand the chest and remain conscious of the kidney area. Soften the kidneys backward. Feel the action of lifting the chest happen closer to the spine than to the skin of the chest. Feel the lift of the chest as an inner lift. Lift the top of the sternum more than the bottom of the sternum.

Tips for lowering the chin. Most importantly remember that the chest comes to meet the chin, not the reverse. With chest maximally expanded extend the chin out and down and then lock the chin onto the notch between the collarbones. It should feel as if you are going to lock onto the sternum. The movement is intentionally exaggerated so that your outward reach through the chin will enable you to lock onto the notch between the collarbones. Once you've caught your lock try to feel a deepening crease or fold between the jaw and chest. As you stay imagine this crease as deepening back and up.

Positioning the head with care. Be aware of keeping the shoulders back and the chest broad. Take care that the weight of the head doesn't cause you to lower it too far forward as this will cause the shoulders to round forward and the chest to fall.

The demeanor and direction of the face. Allow the brain to remain passive. The skin of the face slopes downward. The eyes remain gazing downward as though looking beneath the cheek bones. Use the downward direction of the face to redirect the upward energy of the in-breath downward.

When to apply jalandhara bandha. Begin to maximize your chin lock as you finish filling the lungs. Jalandhara bandha is strongest when the lungs are full. Imagine that you are redirecting the expansive, upward movement of the inhalation (prana vayu) downward as you lock the chin to the chest during inhalation and in the gap when the lungs are filled to capacity.

Receptivity. Use the downward direction of your chin lock to observe the physical and mental feeling of the posture. Do not force or strain, nor allow the mind to become hectic, busy, or heated. Rather, become receptive and cool, relax the brain, and allow the breath's natural power to sweep through you without your doing anything to make it happen. Appreciate the self-generating nature of the breath's rhythm, the continual back and forth sway of the inhalation and exhalation can be likened to a robust, cosmic swing that never winds down.

Reset your position periodically. Occasionally lift your head during exhalation and relieve any built-up strain or tension in the jaw, neck, and shoulders. Return to natural breath if the need to rest and reorient arises, then begin again when ready.

Modifications. Use a rolled towel between your jaw and chest. Reasons for use:
- Your chin doesn't come down onto the chest with ease.
- Your head comes too far forward and down when you attempt the bandha.
- You can't maintain the expansion across the chest when performing the lock.
- You feel tension in the neck, jaw, and upper back area.
- The brain becomes agitated.

If you use a rolled towel do not harden the jaw or clamp down too hard onto the towel. Take frequent breaks and reset the position often.

Jalandhara bandha gesture in a lying down position. Use the supine position to work with the opposing actions that redirect prana vayu downward. Discover support from the ground through the legs by connecting the feet and legs to the wall and ground. These actions make it easier to experience mula bandha action within the pelvis.

References from The Hatha Yoga Pradipika
- At the end of puraka, jalandhara bandha should be performed

and at the end of kumbhaka, and at the beginning of rechaka uddhyana bandha should be performed.[1]

· Closing the passages with jalandhara bandha firmly at the end of puraka and expelling the air slowly is called murchha, from its causing the mind to swoon and giving comfort.[2]

· By stopping the throat (by jalandhara bandha) the air is drawn in from the outside and carried. Just as a snake struck with a stick becomes straight like a stick, in the same way, shakti (shushumna) becomes straight at once. Then the kundalini becoming as if it were dead, and, leaving both the of main branching nadis (ida and pingala) enters the shushumna (the middle passage).[3]

· Fill in the air, keeping the chin firm against the chest, and, having pressed in the air, the mind should be fixed on the middle of the eyebrows, or in the shushumna.[4]

References from The Shiva Samhita
· Having contracted the muscles of the throat, press the chin on the breast. The fire in the region of the navel (the gastric juice drinks the nectar which exudes out of the thousand-petaled lotus). Practice jalandhara in order to prevent the nectar from being consumed.[5]

---

1   *The Hatha Yoga Pradipika* II–45
2   *The Hatha Yoga Pradipika* II–69
3   *The Hatha Yoga Pradipika* III–11,12
4   *The Hatha Yoga Pradipika* III–20
5   *The Yoga Samhita* IV–38

Jalandhara Bandha Gesture

The physical act of locking the chin to the top of the chest commonly leads to improper positioning of the head, neck, upper back, and chest areas. For this reason the sadhaka can make use of the gesture of jalandhara bandha instead of the actual lock in order to energetically simulate the lock without completing the physical action of doing it. The meditative gesture is a downward look into the torso, a marvelous view of the expansive upward direction of the inhalation, an inward containment of pranic energy, and a redirection of upward energy downward.

Use the gesture as a way of familiarizing yourself with the muscular-skeletal actions of the lock as you are learning pranayama. And also apply the gesture if your head, neck, shoulders, and upper back restrict your movement and thus prevent you from properly performing the actions of the lock.

Extra Notes

- The yogi contemplates the great energetic breathing event that calls for an equally great counter energetic event, the chin lock. He understands why jalandhara has a foremost place in the heart of a yogi and in the sacred texts, and he appreciates its widespread fame and longevity.

- The yogi uses his imagination to create jalandhara and not only the physical action. He uses body and mind to define the role of the chin lock in redirecting the upward direction of prana vayu downward.

- Through applying the chin lock along with the other two major bandhas (mula and uddhyana) the aspirant endeavors to direct awareness exclusively into the middle axis during pranayama.

Mula Bandha

Mula: root, foundation, first basis, earth.
Bandha: redirect, stop, close, lock.

Mula bandha is the root lock by which you contract and seal the pelvic floor, thereby stopping the downward energetic pattern of the out-breath (apana). It is an important yoga technique for directing energy (prana) within the nadis (channels) that make up the subtle body (pranamaya kosha).

Mula bandha's physical action is said to isolate, contract, and lift the pelvic floor center (called the perineal body). But this is an extremely challenging action to perform, and thus it can be helpful to know the three following practices within the pelvic floor area:

(1) Ashvini mudra (contracting the anus).

(2) Mula bandha (contracting the perineal body).

(3) Vajroli mudra (contracting the urogenital area).

Mula bandha can have different meanings, locations, and applications, and at times all three of the above-listed contractions (ashvini, mula, vajroli) in varying combinations can be different names for mula bandha. The exact physical location of mula bandha can change with the changes in the alignment of the pelvis that come as result of adopting different asanas.

For the purposes of working with mula bandha during the breathing exercises in the video series, *A Guide to Ujjayi Breathing*, I suggest that you:

- Contract the entire pelvic floor as means of starting to understand how to activate mula bandha.

- Mentally divide the diamond shape of the pelvic floor into two triangles whose points face away from each other. You will then have a front or urogenital triangle whose point is the pubic bone and a back or anal triangle whose point is the coccyx. The two triangles will share a common base, a transverse line that divides the pelvic floor evenly in half. Anatomically the middle point in this line is called the central tendon and is the location of the perineal body, the place you attempt to isolate your contraction to activate mula bandha. You can then begin to work with each of the three practices (ashvini, vajroli, and mula bandha), either separately or in combination.

For example, you can work to isolate each triangle individually. Attempt to contract the back triangle, the anal region, ashwini. Ashwini might be the easiest of the three areas to contract. Guruji said that mula bandha is a contraction of the anus. *The Hatha Yoga Pradipika* says, "This mula bandha is spoken of by the yogis as done by contracting the anus."[1]

Next work to contract the front triangle, attempt to isolate the vajroli mudra, urogenital area.

- Finally, focus your awareness in the middle between ashwini and vajroli, attempt to clarify and isolate your lift of the perineal body that runs across the center of the pelvic floor. Aim to isolate the contraction in the center even though you may involuntarily recruit muscles from other areas.

The pelvic basin. The arrangement of bones that make up the pelvic bowl comprise the two pelvic halves that are joined together in the back by the sacrum and coccyx and in the front by the pubic symphysis (pubic bone). The coccyx and pubic bone along with the sitting bones are the bones that form the bottom of this pelvic basin, and they are also the bones that form the bony boundaries of the floor of the pelvis.

Details of the pelvic floor. Diamond shaped whose four bony corners are: 1, pubic bone; 2, coccyx; 3 and 4, the two sitting bones.

---

1   *The Hatha Yoga Pradipika* III–61

Energetic Concepts of Mula Bandha

Your work with the pelvic floor is more than a physical practice of contracting certain muscles in the lower pelvis. Whether you contract the anus, genitals, or the perineum, it is more valuable to focus on mula bandha as an energetic redirection of apana vayu from downward to upward. *The Shiva Samhita* says, "Pressing well the anus with the heel, forcibly draw upward the apana vayu slowly by practice."[1] And in *The Serpent Power*, John Woodroffe said, "The natural course of apana is downward, but by a contraction at muladhara it is made to go upward through the shushumna where it meets prana."[2]

Through the practice of mula bandha you set up the conditions for accessing the contents of your mind. Placing your awareness within your pelvis you cultivate the experience of the perineal space as the source of immovable asanas, subtle inward discernment, and sacred internal worship and communion. And paradoxically to access the imaginal, psychological, emotional, and unconscious parts of your psyche, you work in a decidedly physical manner with asanas and pranayama; curiously orienting your awareness, posture, and movement from within a tiny area inside your pelvis.

The energetic aspect of practicing mula bandha is to seal in your prana in order to withdraw inward so that prana shakti can awaken at the base and enter the tiny middle channel, the glorious, central, vertical conduit. Closing in your prana can be psychologically viewed as an alchemical closing of the vessel, as a decision to create an internal and psychological view of yourself, as a place of contemplation, abidance, analyzation, reflection, healing, and realization through inner awareness where you experience and investigate the contents of your mind.

The psychic vessel that you create within yourself with the help

---

1   *The Shiva Samhita* IV–41
2   *The Serpent Power, Dover Publications (June 1, 1974)*

of mula bandha can give you an animated, slowed-down view of your mind and teach you to observe the psychic contents that present themselves to you without bias or interference. Purifying and concentrating the mind is partly a matter of carefully observing your thoughts, moods, reactions, and emotions. Practice teaches you to struggle with yourself enough to allow this investigative observation to happen routinely. The eventual goal is to allow your mental contents to arise and settle freely without you grabbing onto or pushing away anything. To do this you can envision a larger container for your thoughts, a hermetically sealed psychic vessel that embraces the contents of your mind as naturally as the sky receives the comings and goings of clouds, rain, wind, storms, and the daily, cyclical, magnificently colored sacred arcing journeys of the sun and moon.

But it is essential to appreciate the extent of the challenge it is to live in a perpetual state of samadhi, of perfectly aligned attention; to imitate the sky with your mind and live in continual awareness of the large background; to see the relativity of thought, the ever-changing nature of thought, from the unbiased, large overview; to be in continual equanimity, a state of mental purity, maturity, and lucidity. Painful mental or physical disturbances arise when you lose the wide, sky-like mental orientation, when you narrow your mind, when you clamp down on certain mental contents, when you create obstructions and hold onto certain contents. This can happen suddenly, swiftly, and unconsciously as you are swept away in a flash and carried off into a preset reaction: a well-grooved, often-traveled thinking or behavioral chain that leads to a well-known painful end. Allowing yourself to be triggered into these conditioned responses, to sensations from the senses, allows your mind to rule over you as a petty tyrant, a brutal dictator who knows how to keep you in place.

When you can look within yourself with uncolored, discerning senses, free of desire, you can realize the grandeur of no mind, the vast, sky quality of consciousness, the pure, reflective capacity of a subtle mind, the invisible, unknowable background, and support to small, ordinary thought.

Deciding to make a serious study of mula bandha can be challenging because of the delicacy of musculature in this area. Perhaps even moreso because there can be a sensitivity in working with the pelvic, genital, and anal areas of the body. I sometimes think of the lower pelvic region as an uncharted dark forest, a wild area, a potential source of fear and tension, a psychologically dangerous and taboo area.

The pelvis houses your sexual energy and the energy behind the fight or flight urge to survive. In their unchecked raw forms these energies have incredible strength and power. It could be said that the way you learn to utilize these energies within you plays a significant role in determining whether you become a fulfilled, creative, well-adjusted person or not. Your sexual energies and/or your emotional energies can become blocked, suppressed, repressed, or expressed without proper control or reflection, and thus cause pain for you and others. Mula bandha is the technique by which you make it a practice to consciously know, harness, and direct the sexual and emotional drives within your core. You endeavor to eliminate the destructive, ego-centered behaviors that these energies can evoke if they remain unconscious, unreflected upon, or carelessly unchecked.

The practice of mula bandha gives you a new and different means of sealing in the energetic life forces within your body so that you can investigate and enter into a relationship with them. You can know how you feel in your loins and guts about all things that enter into your world—people, places, experiences. And instead of blind or instinctual, reaction you learn to make careful choices based on self-reflection and analysis. You decide how or whether to express or check the energy behind your feelings. You must know and interact with your powerful emotional drives to establish a strong basis for emotional health and stability, and to find a soulful means of personal creative expression. You attain yoga, self-knowledge, in part by learning how to trust, respond to and express your feelings and your sexuality.

Mula bandha teaches you not to fear the forces and energies within you, not to be a helpless victim of the energy that drives your unconscious depths. It teaches you to let go of shame and guilt around your sexuality, anger, and envy, and to respect the deep primal energies within you; to trust, harness, and celebrate the power of these drives. Yoga practice helps you learn to follow their wisdom and their dictates consciously, creatively, and constructively. Utilizing mula bandha to become emotionally and sexually mature can be the main source of freeing and harnessing your life force, prana, and attaining success in pranayama.

Using your physical practice to access your deep psychology is facilitated by imagining a change of location for your mind. Instead of thinking with your head, move energetically down and think from your center. Allow the physical experience of your feelings to resonate from a deep source within your belly. Thus discernment, movement, and awareness will come from a more sensual, intuitional, bodily place instead of a heady, intellectual place that is removed from your center.

Decisions about movement, postural alignment, or emotional reactions that come from your head have an entirely different quality than choices that originate consciously within your guts and loins. Awakening mula bandha is about allowing yourself to embody the authentic, unmasked energies within you, energies that reveal how you truly feel.

Seen in this light, you can appreciate the potency of the practice of pranayama where you endeavor to strike a single immovable seat and use your breath to churn and stir up your prana, and then harness, control, and direct it. You purposely activate your feelings, your sexuality, and all the deepest, most powerful energetic forces within you. You endeavor to put all of your prana into circulation, to light up the entire network of energetic circuitry within you. You use the sword of discrimination to scan through the full extent of your inner-world lighting—even the most stubbornly dark, unconscious energies. Accepting and transforming such unlit, obstructed areas is one major theme in practice. Such obstructions can be physical, psychological, emotional, or behavioral. They can be resistant to direction, and automatically flow in certain fixed ways, or remain stubbornly stuck and unmovable.

By helping you clean through and free the energy that flows in the nadis, your yoga practice helps you make a complete investigation. You look within with full courage. Your passion is to know and see everything that is within you with an eye toward love, acceptance, compassion, mercy, and joy. By sincerely practicing the eight limbs you are perfected; you come into right relationship with yourself. Practice helps you find an ongoing, sacred, messy inward celebration that smiles upon and lessens your flaws, failures, crookedness, and ignorance. You give up fear, and you trust that through grace and effort you will come to self-knowledge and self-love in your own way and on your own terms. Apply yourself to mula bandha during kumbhaka and fully embrace your shakti, the energy of your depths.

Your Initiation Into Mula Bandha in Three Steps

In pranayama practice you adopt a single seat to conduct your study of the breathing patterns of the prana and apana vayus and to study kumbhaka, retention, the suspended breath that forms a gap between the vayu patterns. Your chosen immovable spot provides the perfect setting for exploring the role of the pelvic floor and mula bandha in pranayama, the perfect setting for receiving your initiation into mula bandha, into its more subtle, energetic, esoteric, and psychologically potent aspects.

The mula bandha initiation involves three steps. Step one is an acknowledgment of the pelvic floor as more than a physical, anatomical part of the body; it is instead a new, important, mysterious, and sacred location within you. It is a central location close to the ground, a sacred seat of awareness, a resting place, a source of vitality and support known as muladhara, the root support. Seeing the pelvic floor in this new light is key to learning how to make the most of the technique of mula bandha.

In step two, you establish a downward apanic connection to the earth. This earth connection can be felt at first as a general rootedness through the lower trunk, lower spine, abdomen, pelvis, and legs. You imagine your seat as wonderfully apanic, heavy, stable, deeply grounded, rooted into the earth. And then you transfer this broad feeling of rootedness to the much smaller, finer, more subtle area of the pelvic floor, and begin to work with the feeling of a deeply rooted connection to the ground from a central point within your lower pelvis. Imagining the downward force of gravity as a persistent, benevolent force that pulls your body toward the earth's center can help you understand the apanic force of rootedness. Apana is complementary to the downward directional pull of gravity, and this is the first part of understanding mula bandha.

Step three of the initiation is in experiencing the activation of an opposite upward direction to the apanic force that occurs in response to your well-established downward connection to the earth. The presence of the downward pull of gravity and of apana vayu within muladhara precipitates the activation of mula bandha, the upward rebound, the dynamic oppositional response to the strength of the downward force.

Your initiation into mula bandha is complete when you attain darduri siddhi, frog leap power! Associating the practice of mula bandha with the powerful buoyant leap of a frog gives you a tangible image for how to energetically experience the combination of the second and third steps of mula bandha. Activating mula bandha involves creating opposite directions of energetic forces within the pelvis, beginning with a powerful, grounded connection to the earth, followed by a corresponding extraordinary feeling of lightness, a rebound, a natural counter response that carries subtle, internal, core energy away from the earth, up through the thin, dynamic, central and vertical channel. The dynamism of mula bandha is like a crouch and spring, a subtle, esoteric, mystical frog leap. Attaining darduri siddhi can serve you well during pranayama by helping you sit still, and yet dynamically settled and buoyant.

Khecari Mudra

Kha: void, space, emptiness.
Cara: moves in, walks in, vehicle of.
Mudra: seal, stamp.

Khecari mudra is a highly revered esoteric practice that is spoken of at length in the sacred texts of hatha yoga. It is known as the best of all mudras,[1] and it is said that all other mudras derive from khecari.[2] However, there is an important point that needs to be cleared up in undertaking this mudra. Khecari is performed by curling the tongue back in mouth far enough to close off the air hole at the back of the throat. This action is said to give the yogi access to the nectar that continuously drips down from an esoteric lake located at the base of the thousand-petaled lotus chakra at the crown. It is traditionally taught that to be able do this requires a long, slow, painful process of cutting the tendon (called the frenulum) beneath the tongue in order to win enough extra mobility to curl the tongue and reach it far enough back to close off the air hole at the back of the palate. However, this potentially dangerous practice is not recommended, nor is it necessary in order to work with the far more practical and safe concept or image of khecari. You can get a similar effect from learning a gentler, less invasive khecari mudra gesture. The gesture is simple and complements ujjayi breathing. The gesture is performed by touching the middle part of the tongue (not the tip or sides) lightly against the palate somewhere behind the teeth. The khecari mudra gesture creates a physical connection between the tongue and palate, an energetic seal that simulates khecari mudra (without cutting the frenulum).

Khecari's value is found in the meditative awareness that comes from contemplating the sacred area called the root of the palate located above the roof of the mouth and below

---

1   *The Shiva Samhita* IV–37
2   *The Shiva Samhita* IV–32

the floor of the brain within the head. Specific locations in the body, such as the root of the palate location of khecari mudra, become sacred because they have an extra capacity to help the poised yogi to direct her consciousness inward. Locating these sacred places within and fixing the mind there happens naturally and spontaneously as a result of serious yoga practice. These inner temple spots are the power places where your consciousness is meant to dwell in order to awaken kinesthetic intelligence and meditation.

Khecari mudra is one of the most important images for improving breathing, postural alignment, and inducing meditative states of refined awareness. Working with the image of cultivating a discerning, awake palate helps you to understand how to align your head and brain in asana and pranayama practice.

The lake of nectar, located at the base of the thousand-petaled lotus, provides the ambrosial beverage coveted by even the gods. Unconsciousness results in the nectar going downward unnoticed where it is wasted and burnt up in the digestive fire in the belly area (manipura). On the other hand awakening the discerning palate through performing khecari mudra is said to help you receive and appreciate the steady, slow supply of this best of beverages.

The powerful image of this lake and its rain of nectar points to the value of contemplating the root of palate. This image can bring you into better postural alignment and lead to subtle, fine, and delicate inner awareness. This image also serves to balance the some of the imbalances that are inherent to learning pranayama. Strain in the head, face, eyes, ears, neck, jaw, and upper back commonly results from applying yourself to the many challenges of learning pranayama. It is all too common to use too much tension producing force as you attempt to concentrate, to prolong your breath, and to increase the duration of your retentions. It is easy for the ego to get caught up in the process, and using khecari mudra can reduce tension and wrongful striving.

- When the skillful Yogi, by placing the tongue at the root of the palate, can crank up the Prana Vayu, then there occurs complete dissolution of all yogas.[1]

- There is a nectar rayed moon, in its proper place on the top of the spinal cord… this faces downward and rains nectar day and night.[2]

- Pointing the tongue upward, when the Yogi can drink the nectar flowing from the moon (situated between the eyebrows) within a month he will certainly conquer death.[3]

- When having firmly closed the glottis by the proper yogic method and contemplating on the goddess Kundalini he drinks (the moon fluid of immortality) he becomes a sage or poet within six months.[4]

- …placing the tongue upward the wise yogi drinks the fluid very slowly…[5]

- The person never dies who contemplates by (way of) pressing the tongue (against the palate), combined with the vital fluid of prana.[6]

- Having conquered all the elements, and being void of all hopes and worldly connections, when the Yogi sitting in the Padmasana, fixes his gaze on the tip of his nose his mind becomes dead and he obtains the spiritual power

---

1   The Shiva Samhita IV–69
2   The Shiva Samhita II–6, 7
3   The Shiva Samhita III–72
4   The Shiva Samhita III–73
5   The Shiva Samhita III–76
6   The Shiva Samhita III–80

called Khecari.[1]

- One who contemplates Anahata, the heart center, obtains the power known as Khecari.[2]

- From the base or the root of the palate, the shushumna extends downward, till it reaches the Muladhar and the perineum.[3]

- And from the heart—the bedrock of the universe—rises the axis of kundalini. Thus the creeping, subterranean, obscure energy shoots up, and like an immobile and vibrant pillar piercing its way through space, it roots the sky in the earth. Then, as khecari, it soars up and roams with total freedom in the infinite firmament of Consciousness.[4]

1 *The Shiva Samhita* V–49
2 *Source Unknown*
3 *The Shiva Samhita* V–121
4 *Kundalini Energy Of The Depths,* by LIlian Silburn

Thoughts On Shushumna

Shushumna: most glorious, the main pranic channel located along the central axis of the body.

Shushumna is the most important image of the entire set of images that make up the internal maps of hatha yoga. By following these maps you will make swift and sure progress in practice. By contemplating the images you can explore specific internal spaces within your body that help you to clear your mind and create states of subtle, refined awareness. You use your asanas and breathing to concentrate your mind, to stubbornly cultivate a steady, unwavering mind that is able to contemplate these inmost, central sacred images. The images come from the sacred texts and can be thought of as aids to help you learn to map your internal world.

Shushumna, thin as a spider's thread, and brilliant as the light of ten million moons, is the most important of these internal images because it is the central and foremost nadi, or pranic channel, that spans the vertical axis between the pelvic floor and the crown of the head.

Shushumna is known as the conduit. It is the vessel that transports awakened kundalini shakti, the coiled, serpentine energy from your depths, to the symbolic thousand-petaled lotus at the crown of the head. The visualization of shushumna helps you to align your asanas, settle into the rhythm of breathing, and activate the three main bandhas that are situated along its central axis. The contemplation of this most glorious axis leads to a clearing of the nadis and a freeing of the life force within you. You then apply subtle action to your bandhas, direct your energy more consciously, attain mind control, and withdraw into the inmost part of the middle channel. There you sip the rare nectar of pure consciousness at the centerless center.

Additional thoughts on Shushumna:
- Highly celebrated and revered shushumna has many names:

Most Glorious, the Median Way, the Middle Channel, the World Mountain, Emptiness, the Void, the Pillar of Light, the Pillar of Fire, the Royal Road, the Middle Road, the Central Pranic Axis, the Central Axis, the Middle Axis.

- The movement of shakti upward is first made possible by the vigorous churning of the breath. The strong breathing actions are achieved by following the breath to its endpoint at the base of the pelvis (out-breath) and to the top of the chest (in-breath). The yogi awakens kundalini by awakening his breath. He uses ujjayi sound in breathing to define and amplify the vayu patterns that accompany the in- and out-breaths. By these best means he suspends his awareness in the middle between the two patterns and enters shushumna.

- By organizing the body and concentrating the mind along the central line, the yogi meditates on his own body as a yantra, a visual instrument of protection, healing, and sattvic buddhi (clarified intellect).

- Concentrating on the vertical axis improves skeletal alignment and provides the wise yogi with a means of skillfully and intelligently performing any asana.

- The aspirant realizes the esoteric implications of shushumna. She contemplates the symbolic reunion of Shakti and Shiva that happens within the subtle core of her body. She then finds within herself a nest, a place of personal refuge and safety, and she withdraws to that internal place during practice.

- Through mapping shushumna she locates herself at the symbolic center of the cosmos, her spinal column becomes the world mountain, her vertical axis supports and upholds all of existence and she becomes the cosmic person.

- Through breathing well in her asana practice, the yogi churns her vital energy. She awakens the dormant spiritual power in her depths and plugs into the hidden, elusive source of energy that lights up the vertical axis (shushumna), infusing the entire body with dynamism and intelligence.

• To live without adequately breathing, without inner awareness, without continual self reflection, without willingness to change, without dharma (spiritual purpose), clogs the nadis and creates energetic knots within the body. Obstructed nadis symbolize the state of suffering experienced by the confused yogi. His unsteady thoughts and erratic behaviors awaken the strong activity of the kleshas (the root causes of pain) within him. The kleshas are avidya (not able to see spiritual truth), followed by asmita (egoism), raga (craving for pleasure), dvesa (aversion to displeasure), and abhinvesha (clinging to life, fear of death). Therefore the practice of asana and pranayama is prescribed in order to purify the nadis and to lessen the strength of the kleshas.

• The confinement of awareness and breath in the middle channel becomes samadhi, perfect inward absorption, here, within shushumna, the yogi enjoys cessation of the irregular movements of thought.

• Repeatedly recalling the visual image of shakti traveling up the glorious axis helps the yogi understand how to perfect his inward absorption, to realize the full extent to which his consciousness can awaken and become absorbed within the depths of his body.

• The yogi learns to see the breath as interiorized prana and shushumna in the form of a tiny, hollow tube, thin as a lotus filament, whose purpose is to carry prana from the inward core upward, through a series of energetic wheels (chakras) to the thousand-petaled lotus at the crown.

• Within shushumna, the yogi is no longer thrown off by the dvandvas' conflicting, oppositional forces. Learning to direct the vayu patterns of prana and apana helps the yogi still the body in asana, and then train his awareness exclusively onto the subtlest rhythmic movements of the vayu breathing patterns. In this way he becomes absorbed within the innermost refuge, shushumna.

- In the beginning Kundalini sleeps at the base of shushumna. Her slumber symbolizes the latent, inactive energy within the uninitiated yogi. The spark that is activated by enthusiasm for practice begins the process of energetic awakening that will unlock latent energy and eventually lead to fulfillment of the yogi's dharma (true purpose).

- For the discerning yogi the practice of asana and pranayama becomes a continual endeavor to orient her physical and mental awareness on the breathing cycle without fear, bias, or judgment. Through this work the aspirant becomes skilled in centering herself; she knows her body, achieves an inner intimacy; she wins a clarity about the contents of her mind and thus enjoys all the fruits of contemplating shushumna.

- Knowledge of shushumna helps the aspirant to develop intelligence of the body that is born of keen inward perception, feeling, and intuition. Making use of this body knowledge, he skillfully performs the postures with animal dexterity and graceful ease. Through knowing the center line, he knows how to align and inhabit his body with poise and awareness.

- Pranayama that is focused on breathing within the middle channel leads the aspiring yogi to a special kind of physical, intuitive body knowledge, an awareness of his singular participation in nature's subtle, continual, comprehensive, and immediate dance.

- By orienting himself along the central plumb line of the body, the yogi learns to size up his inner states swiftly; indeed, he responds with an immediacy born of intuitive certainty. In *The Yoga Sutras*, meditation born of such immediacy and totality of comprehension is called pratibha, a sudden flash of illumination. The yogi makes a deft internal scan, a skillful sweep of awareness that brings alignment to his body and truth to his mental orientation. His skill helps him accomplish the awakening of kundalini in an instant.

- The nadis are nearly infinite in number, and within the body they form a vast network of riverbed-like channels that branch and subdivide; they reach from the central core to the farthest limits of the interior spaces of the body. Part of the work with the nadis is purification; when they are clear and unobstructed these nadis conduct life force throughout the body and allow for a concentration of prana within the middle channel that leads to the experience of samadhi, cognitive absorption, ashtanga's eighth limb.

- To awaken shushumna nadi is to come to trust the breath and the body, and that is how the accomplished yogi comes to listen to his inward-directed consciousness. He knows the benefits of breathing with thoroughness and precision, and therefore when simply breathing he attains total absorption, he enjoys the involvement of his entire body in his breath, movement, and postures.

References from The Hatha Yoga Pradipika
- ...(if) the breath does not pass through the middle channel (shushumna), owing to the impurities of the nadis, how can then success be attained?[1]

- By drawing up from below (mula bandha) and contracting the throat (jalandhara bandha) and by pulling back the middle of the front portion of the body (uddhyana bandha) the prana goes to the shushumna nadi.[2]

- Kundalini awakens by kumbhaka, and by its awakening,

---

1 *The Hatha Yoga Pradipika* II–4
2 *The Hatha Yoga Pradipika* II–46

shushumna becomes free from impurities.[1]

- Steadiness of mind comes when the air moves freely in the middle. That is the manomani condition, which is attained when the mind becomes calm.[2]

- Shushumna (sunya padavi) becomes a main road for the passage of prana, and the mind then becomes free from all connections (with its objects of enjoyments) and death is then evaded.[3]

- Shushumna, Sunya Padavi, Brahma Randhra, Maha Patha, Smasana, Shambhavi, Madhya Marga, are names of one and the same thing.[4]

- This middle nadi becomes straight by steady practice of asanas, pranayama, and mudras.[5]

- When the prana flows in the shushumna, and the mind has entered shunya, then the yogi is free from the effects of karmas.[6]

- How can it be possible to get knowledge so long as the prana is living and the mind has not died? No one else can get moksha, except one who can make one's prana and mind latent.[7]

- In this body there are 72,000 openings of nadis; of these, the shushumna which has the shambhavi shakti in it, is the only important one, the rest are useless.[8]

- By stopping the throat (jalandhara bandha) the air is drawn

---

1 *The Hatha Yoga Pradipika* II-75
2 *The Hatha Yoga Pradipika* II–42
3 *The Hatha Yoga Pradipika* III–3
4 *The Hatha Yoga Pradipika* III–4
5 *The Hatha Yoga Pradipika* III–117
6 *The Hatha Yoga Pradipika* IV–12
7 *The Hatha Yoga Pradipika* IV–15
8 *The Hatha Yoga Pradipika* IV–18

in from the outside and carried down. Just as a snake struck with a stick becomes straight like a stick, in the same way shushumna, by way of shakti, becomes straight at once.[1]

References from The Shiva Samhita
- Shushumna alone is the highest channel for prana and is beloved by the yogis, other vessels are subordinate to it in the body.[2]

1   *The Hatha Yoga Pradipika* III–10
2   *The Shiva Samhita* II–16

"…only the kumbhaka pranayama, which is purificatory and useful for self realization, is useful."[1]

– Sri K. Pattabhi Jois

---

1   *The Yoga Mala* pg 23

Kumbhaka

The Art of Becoming Void-Minded

The main reason why pranayama is one limb of only eight limbs in ashtanga yoga is because of the role that kumbhaka (breath retention) plays in concentrating awareness and contemplating the mind. Retaining the breath is a principle means of restraining thought, of bringing about the ultimate goal of yoga: "citta vrtti nirodha,"[1] the ceasing of the turnings of thought.

Consider this passage from *The Hatha Yoga Pradipika*:

> Both the mind and breath are united together, like milk and water; and both of them are equal in their activities. Mind begins its activities where there is breath, and the prana begins its activities where there is mind... By the suspension of one, therefore, comes the suspension of the other...[2]

Thus, if to retain the breath is to restrain the mind, then to successfully practice pranayama is to pierce directly through to the heart of yoga, to transcend the activities of the mind. Then also the practice of kumbhaka is less about breath control and more about mental control, about learning to stop the breath as

1 *The Yoga Sutras* I–2
2 *The Hatha Yoga Pradipika* IV–24, 25

a means of learning to stop the incessant activity of the mind.

One definition of the word bandha is to stop. This refers not only to the stopping of prana but also to the stopping of thought. For example during bahya (external) kumbhaka you emphasize uddhyana and mula bandhas in order to seal in apana vayu at your base and confine the prana in the central channel. And during antara (internal) kumbhaka you apply more jalandhara bandha at the throat in order to seal in prana vayu at the top of the chest and further confine prana in the middle. In both cases, by utilizing the main bandhas in varying strengths, you endeavor to seal your prana within the middle channel and to cause the mind to turn away from activity, to withdraw from the pull of outward desires and distracted states, and to concentrate toward spaciousness, internal absorption, and the awakening of buddhi, subtle discernment.

Applying bandhas in combination with kumbhaka helps you to withdraw your attention away from distraction and outer desires.

The Hatha Yoga Pradipika says this:

> There are two causes of the activities of the mind. 1) vasana (desires) and 2) respiration (the movement of prana). Of these the destruction of one is the destruction of both.[1]

By using kumbhaka to stop the breath and applying bandhas to stop the movements of prana, you can cause the destruction of the distracting desires that lead the mind into painful, restless activity and away from the central axis.

The *Yoga Sutras* state that practicing kumbhaka helps you overcome the nine mental obstacles, called antaryas,[2] that can disrupt concentration and thwart meaningful practice. The obstacles disrupt smooth, regular breathing, and cause the mind to become clouded, restless, disturbed (citta vishepah). Practicing kumbhaka clears the mind (citta prasadam), by helping you

---

1   *The Hatha Yoga Pradipika* IV–22
2   *The Yoga Sutras* I–30 through I–34

regularize your breathing and causing the flow of prana to withdraw into the middle channel, known as shunya, empty.

Yoga Sutra I-34
pracchardana-vidhāraṇābhyām vā prāṇasya

Citta the mind field becomes settled, clear when either the in- or out-breath is restrained

Also, *The Yoga Sutras* say that practicing pranayama makes the mind fit for dharana, concentration, the seventh limb,[1] providing another example of withdrawing inward to find the spacious mental clarity and equanimity in the middle.

Yoga Sutra II-53
dhāraṇāsu ca yogyatā manash

Through the practice of pranayama the mind becomes fit for concentration

Mental disturbance is thought of as the opposite of shunya (emptiness), as the result of confusion, of decentralized awareness, of a scattered, undisciplined, antagonistic, discursive, excessively active mind. Ignorance, toxicity, and imbalance are the result of habitually failing to find an internal center, an inability to breathe with a steadiness that helps you locate your awareness in the middle. The opposite of a cluttered, busy, active mind is a spacious, empty, receptive mind.

Through stopping the mind during kumbhaka the mind becomes empty, spacious, vast, disciplined, purified, reflective, absorbed in the middle, receptive, still, and settled. This emptiness partly comes from being free from unwanted, harmful desires and other uneconomical distracted mental states. Practicing kumbhaka gives substance to the image of the healthy mind as imbued with shunya—emptiness, void, or receptivity— and is why the yogi endeavors to become void-minded.

---

1 *The Yoga Sutras* II–53

Through kumbhaka you can experience the relief and the value of no mind that says if the nature of an undisciplined mind is to be engaged in constant pain-causing activity, then the state of no mind, of stopping thought and transcending the mind, will bring a new experience of delight, a more accurate and integrated experience of the splendors of the immediate apprehension of the world. By stopping the breath and stopping thought you win the ability to receive knowledge of what and who the universe is without the imperfect, biased, truth-obscuring colorings of the mind's routine round of pointless activity.

The yoga teachings present the image of the ultimate condition of the mind as Void in many different ways. One way is through the frequent use of the concept of nirodha, of stopping of thought.

Yoga Sutra I-2
yogaś citta-vṛtti-nirodhaḥ

Yoga is the ceasing of the turnings of thought or
Yoga is the stopping of the activity of the mind

This classic sutra becomes more real through stopping your breath. You become more ready to experience nirodha through the practice of kumbhaka.

Another example of the value of shunya within *The Yoga Sutras* comes from the concept of nirbija samadhi,[1] or seedless samadhi. This image communicates that the highest form of internal absorption is when there is concentrative awareness with no seed. This implies that there is no need of support from the pervasive cyclical mental activity that begins with the germination of the seed and continues on endlessly through the cycles of birth, sustenance, and decay.

Nirbija samadhi happens when the mind is empty, pure, accurately and perfectly reflective of its object of concentration. The observer ceases to exist because there is no longer a distinction

---

1 *The Yoga Sutras* I–51

between an observer and an object being observed. There is the realization that the object and the observer of the object are not different. This is the concept of nirodha seen from another angle, the experience of stopping thought seen from another perspective. When the mind

is pure enough to accurately reflect the object of meditation, the activity of thought stops, and there is no longer a need for mental activity to arise, no longer a need to generate mental activity to balance prior activity. In this way all notions are left behind.

Consider this passage from *The Yoga Vasistha* during a conversation between young Ram and his guru Vasistha:

> My son when, in the infinite consciousness, the consciousness becomes aware of itself as its own object, there is the seed of ideation. This is very subtle. But soon it becomes gross and fills the whole space, as it were. When consciousness is engrossed in this ideation it thinks the object is distinct from the subject. Then the ideation begins germinate, and to grow. Ideation multiplies naturally by itself. This leads to sorrow, not to happiness. There is no cause for sorrow in this world other than this ideation.[1]

The practice of kumbhaka can give you a practical, experiential entrance into the most central and important images of yoga's teachings, leading you into the core of practice, into continual receptivity, contemplation, and self-reflection.

The experience of nirodha, of stopping the prana and thus stopping thought, is an experience that leaves language behind.

Consider this passage from *The Hatha Yoga Pradipika*:

> When all the thoughts and activities are destroyed, then the absorbed stage is produced, to describe this stage is beyond the power of speech, and is known only by self-experience alone.[2]

---

1   *The Supreme Yoga; Yoga Vasistha*   pg 134
2   *The Hatha Yoga Pradipika*   IV–32

Tips for improving the quality of your attention in kumbhaka:

- Mudras are internal seals that can help you to reduce the movement of thought within you as you perform kumbhaka.

- Prana, the creative force that hides within the breath, is described as a goddess, Shakti, or Jagadambe, the Mother of all moving things. Meet Shakti by entering into play with her through regulating the breath and attempting to stop her movements. Make use of the breath as your greatest boon; make use of this ready opportunity to encounter the Great Mother, Shakti, in the simple, accessible rhythms of the breath and the gaps between the rhythms.

- Remain undisturbed, mentally equanimous, during kumbhaka. Adopt an agreeable demeanor as you apply intense focus to the suspended gap between breaths.

- Maintain receptivity throughout the body, release tension and strain, and be careful not to agitate your mind by attempting to overextend the length of your retentions.

- Respect your changing capacity for kumbhaka on each given day. Place more value on the quality of awareness during retentions than on the length or number of them.

- Remember to enjoy your breathing in a very basic, primal way. Allow yourself to become benevolently absorbed in the refuge of emptiness and silence within.

- Covet the experience of void that kumbhaka opens to you. Imagine the void as emptiness, as background, as sky, as vast enough to contain, swallow, and absorb the activity of your mind.

- Use bandhas to stop the movements of prana and as a means of improving the quality of your awareness while performing kumbhaka.

- Stopping the breath leads to musings about the experience of consciousness beyond thought. This leads to images of void, of shunya, of emptiness. Develop the experience of yoga by contemplating these profound images. Allow these images to transform your experience of the physical body, to help you locate your center within the pelvis, and thus to transform the experience of the location of the mind inside the body.

- In the yoga teachings the goal to stop thought comes from associating thought with the concepts of karma, samskara, and kleshas. Nirodha comes from realizing the necessity to stop the mind's activity.

"Man is composed of such elements as vital breath, deeds, thought, and the senses—all of them deriving their being from the Self."[1]

– The Prasna Upanishad (Prasnopanishad)

---

1   *The Upanishads, Breath of The Eternal*   pg 34

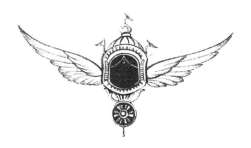

Stories

Remembering the Source

One time within the ongoing battle for supremacy between the gods and the demons, the gods won a great victory over the demons. The gods congratulated themselves and took all the credit for winning when actually it was Brahman, the great invisible spirit, who caused them to win. Deciding to teach the gods a lesson, Brahman appeared before them in disguise. On seeing the stranger they talked among themselves saying:

"Who is that stranger?"

"I don't know."

"One of us should go over there and talk to him to try to figure out who he is."

They sent Agni, the god of fire (tapas), to find who the stranger was. Agni approached him.

Stranger: "Who are you?"

Agni: "You have probably heard of me, I am Agni the god of fire."

Stranger: "Ah… and what do you do?"

Agni: "I am fierce, that I can burn anything in the three worlds."

The stranger placed a tiny, piece of dry straw on the ground in front of Agni and said, "Burn this."

Agni tried with all his might to burn the little piece of straw and nothing happened. He returned to the other gods no closer to discovering who the stranger was.

Next they sent Vayu, the wind god (of breath), to find out the stranger's identity.

Stranger: "And who are you?"

Vayu: "I am known as Vayu, the great god of the wind, my strength is renowned. I can blow away anything in existence."

The stranger placed a tiny piece of dried straw before Vayu and said, "Blow this piece of straw away."

Vayu blew and he blew but he couldn't move the piece of straw.

The gods then sent Indra to investigate, but when Indra approached the stranger suddenly vanished, and in his place stood Durga the great Goddess. Indra asked Durga who the stranger was. She laughed and scolded him saying: "That was the Great Invisible Spirit come to have some sport with you. You gods didn't cause your victory, Brahman caused it and you were over-eager to take credit. Brahman came to toy with you a bit so that you would see your folly and learn from it."

The gods were humbled in realizing their mistake but also doubly blessed in that they were credited with coming into close proximity to the Great Invisible Spirit, close to catching a glimpse of the mysterious, elusive Brahman, even though they didn't succeed in guessing who he was.

This story from the *Kenopanishad* (*The Kena Upanishad*) reminds the yogi that he practices to remember the nameless one who is behind the fire, the breath, the sensations. The friend is difficult to know, and yet to attempt to know the ultimate invisible source of all is the highest aim of practice. And pranayama is a diving down into the depths of the inward ocean like a free diver who dives unencumbered, without even an oxygen tank. The inward-minded yogi suspends his breath. He stops the rhythmic movements of the vayu patterns, and during the span of time that exists in that gap between breaths he humbly surrenders; he lowers his head to Brahman, the unknowable, the source of the sacred knowledge found within. The yogi remembers that his progress, and his victory, are the gifts of this secret one who is the unseen, unknown cause behind everything.

This is true even though these three, Agni, Vayu, and Indra, are the yogi's most trustworthy and important allies in the practice of pranayama. Agni represents tapas, the internal heat of the sacrificial fire, the heat of the effort to regulate the breath and to steady the bucking mind. Vayu, the element air, represents the profound aspect of breath: breath that becomes prana when interiorized through inward absorption and performing the various pranayama techniques. And Indra represents the senses and sense organs that the yogi endeavors to redirect from outward to inward through breathing and stopping his breath.

The wise yogi perceives these three helpers as living energies within himself, the inner fire, the subtle breath, and the absorbed senses. The importance of these three gods of pranayama is clear and evident. The wise yogi also remembers that each yoga technique is not an end in itself; it's not just fire for fire's sake, or experiencing sensations for the gross pleasures they offer. Rather, the yogi cultivates fire to better conduct the hunt for the elusive secret one who is behind the techniques. He observes his sensations in order to glean their subtle, profound aspect, to understand and attain their source. He practices breath control, ujjayi, viloma, and kumbhaka to share the tiniest moment of communion with the friend.

Prana Is First and Foremost

Once upon a time the ten senses (five jnanendriyas: seeing, feeling, tasting, hearing, and smelling; and five karmendriyas: walking, grasping, speaking, procreating, eliminating) and the prana inside the body were having a discussion, and an argument arose concerning who among them was the most important personage within the body. Each of the senses claimed that he was the most important, the eyes pointed out the importance of the power of seeing, the ears of hearing, the feet of walking, and so forth.

The prana listened for some time with a stern, sly, twinkle in his eye, and finally made his opinion known by getting up and making as if to leave the body, and involuntarily all the others arose at the same time to leave with him like drone bees following their queen. The prana sat back down and everyone acknowledged that prana alone is greatest because everything else within the body is dependent on him for life. The body and the person can thrive without seeing or hearing but not without prana, not without the animating force, the secret, hidden source of all creative activity.

Quotes from the Prasnopanishad (The Prasna Upanishad)
- As spokes in the nave of a wheel, everything in the universe, mantras, songs, all dynamic activities, all spiritual endeavors, are fixed in the prana.[1]

- Oh Prana! Make my body auspicious, you abide in speech, in the ear, in the eye, you pervade the mind. Please do not go away.[2]

- You (Prana) are the true dynamic principle behind the senses, which are the chief factors of the body.[3]

---

1 *Prasnopanishad (The Prasna Upanishad)* Query II–6
2 *Prasnopanishad (The Prasna Upanishad)* Query II–12
3 *Prasnopanishad (The Prasna Upanishad)* Query II–8

- This (Prana) burns as fire, shines like the sun, rains as cloud, rules like Indra. This bright one is the wind (breath), it is the earth, it is all matter. It is that which has form and that which is formless, and also what is eternal.[1]

Part of attaining vayu siddhi is to perceive prana everywhere and in everything and thus to be able to receive nourishing energy not only from food and drink, but from postures; breath; consciousness; relationship; the sun; earth and sky; creativity and love.

The yogi learns to refine his power to direct the flow of energy within himself. Seeing the basic force that animates all manifestation as the same force that creates all the vital processes within his body, the activities of his senses and his mind, the yogi learns to see the connection between himself and the entirety, between his small but essential discovery of truth within himself and the universal power of truth to create miraculous transformation.

When he practices pranayama he aims to master his prana, to direct his mind at will. He yokes his awareness to his breath and thus concentrates his mind. He ends his tendency to allow his mind to flow toward reality-obscuring and pain-causing activity. He leads his thoughts away from the nonessential and toward unbias, toward a middle place of nonactivity and rest. This knowledge helps the yogi tap the unlimited pranic power of the Self that lives within him. He becomes like Hanuman who is known as Maha Veer, the one with great vitality.

Profound meditation that is the result of asana and pranayama practice reveals that prana is the great source, the nourisher, the energy that enables a person to walk through the stages of inner evolution to individuation and to reach the finest human essence.

---

1 *Prasnopanishad (The Prasna Upanishad)* Query II–5

"Through the practice of pranayama the mind becomes arrested in a single direction and follows the movement of the breath."[1]

– Sri K. Pattabhi Jois

---

1   *Yoga Mala* pg 23

The Ashtanga
Pranayama Sequence

The Practice List

Here, you will find an itemized list of the five pranayama's that make up the ashtanga yoga pranayama sequence as offered in the video series, *A Guide to the Pranayama Sequence*. Note: the term control means kumbhaka (retention).

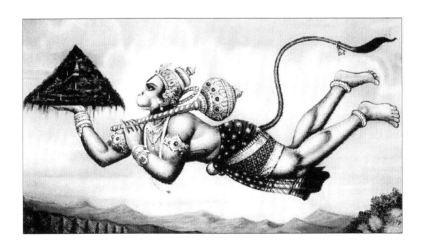

Pranayama #1: Ujjayi
Parts A and B

To begin: *3 breaths*

Part A

(1) Exhale, control (retention)
(2) Inhale
   Repeat steps 1 and 2 three times
   Transition to step 3 with no extra breaths

(3) Inhale, control (retention)
(4) Exhale
   Repeat steps 3 and 4 three times

   3 breaths

Part B

(1) Inhale, control
(2) Exhale, control
   Repeat steps 1 and 2 three times

   3 breaths

Pranayama #2: Nadi Shodana
Parts A and B

Part A—Sama Vrtti (same action)

Take vishnu mudra
Inhale both nostrils
Exhale left

(1) Inhale right, control
(2) Exhale left, control
(3) Inhale left, control
(4) Exhale right, control
Repeat steps 1 through 4 three times

Part B—Visama Vrtti (irregular action)

Transition to Part B with no extra breaths
(1) Inhale right, control
(2) Exhale right, control

Repeat steps 1 through 2 two times

Transition
Inhale right, control
Exhale left, control

(1) Inhale left, control
(2) Exhale left, control
Repeat steps 1 through 2 three times

Transition
Inhale left, control
Exhale right, control
Inhale right
Exhale left
Release vishnu mudra

3 breaths

Pranayama #3: Bhastrika

(1) Inhale
(2) Exhale and inhale, perform bhastrika
continuously for up to one minute
(3) Exhale
(4) Inhale, control
(5) Exhale
Repeat steps 1 through 5 three times

3 breaths

Pranayama #4: Surya and Chandra Bhedana

Take vishnu mudra
Inhale both nostrils
Exhale left

(1) Inhale right, control
(2) Exhale left
Repeat steps 1 and 2 three times

(3) Inhale left, control
(4) Exhale right
Repeat steps 3 and 4 three times

Inhale right
Exhale left
Release vishnu mudra

3 breaths

Pranayama #5: Sitali

(1) Inhale while performing sitali, control
(2) Exhale
   Repeat steps 1 through 2 three times

   3 breaths

Instructions for the Five Pranayamas

Here, you will find detailed instructions for each of the five pranayamas in the ashtanga yoga pranayama sequence.

Pranayama #1—Ujjayi
With Bahya and Antara Kumbhakas

Uj: upward, expansive.
Jaya: victorious.
Bahya: external.
Antara: internal.
Kumbhaka: retention.

Sri K. Pattabhi Jois called ujjayi breathing simply breathing with sound. Ujjayi is the foundational pranayama technique that is used in conjunction with virtually all other pranayama techniques. Use ujjayi breathing between sections and when working with the exercises in the video series, *A Guide to the Pranayama Sequence*. This first pranayama also introduces bahya kumbhaka (retention after exhaling) and antara kumbhaka (retention after inhaling). The kumbhaka ratio is approximately 6:4 inhalation/exhalation. This means that if you retain the in-breath for 20 seconds you will retain the out-breath for 14 or 15 seconds. It is natural and logical to retain the breath for a longer duration after inhalation than after exhalation. And this indicates that achieving the proper ratio sorts itself out if you follow the guideline of not forcing your retentions. (For more teachings on ujjayi breathing see the introductory materials in the video series, *A Guide to Ujjayi Breathing* and the "Ujjayi Breathing" section beginning on page 41 of this book.)

Pranayama #2—Nadi Shodana

Nadi: channel, tube, circulatory vessel.
Shodana: cleanse, purify.

Nadi shodana (cleansing of pranic channels). Developing skill in the technique of nadi shodana is necessary in order to understand the unique language and purpose of pranayama. Within the body, prana, life force, flows through circulatory channels called nadis that spread throughout the body resembling a giant inverted tree with a vast network of branching tributaries and an inverted root network.

The first, most central nadi is known as shushumna. Next in order of importance are a pair of nadis known as ida and pingala, and they are associated with the left and right nostrils, respectively. The sacred texts on hatha yoga state that there can be no success in yoga if the nadis remain clogged or obstructed, and this is why the concept of purifying the nadis through pranayama and other yoga techniques is prescribed. Thus, by practicing pranayama daily, you invigorate and purify your bodily systems by performing nadi shodana with kumbhaka.

The second pranayama introduces digital pranayama also known as alternate nostril breathing. (See instructions for vishnu mudra hand positioning in the video series, *A Guide to the Pranayama Sequence.*)

Working with the technique of nadi shodana gives the discerning yogi an elementary means of regulating his prana. By manipulating the flow of breath through ida and pingala, he learns to direct prana's movements into shushumna. The repeated practice of nadi shodana and the other pranayama techniques helps the wise yogi attain vayu siddhi; he wins mastery of the movements of prana within his body, and thus is able to confine his prana in the middle channel.

Pranayama #3—Bhastrika

Bhastrika: bellows.

Bhastrika is a highly active, energy-rousing technique that tones the abdomen and helps you to activate your respiratory musculature. The forceful rhythmic pumping of the breath churns the belly and stirs up the dormant, sluggish energy within muladhara, the root support chakra at the base. Kundalini shakti, the coiled pranic energy within muladhara, is awakened and summoned to enter the middle channel.

To practice this pranayama technique you imitate the rhythmic pumping action of a blacksmith's bellows (hence the name) by rapidly contracting and releasing your abdomen and performing a long series of staccato, forced exhalations followed by immediate, reflexive inhalations.

Bhastrika is also one of the shat (six) kriyas (cleansings) that are well known, important purifying practices in classic hatha yoga, and this points to its digestive cleansing benefits. When following along with the video, it may take time to develop enough skill, strength, and/or stamina to perform bhastrika breathing for the full duration of the repetitions as presented in the video series, *A Guide to the Pranayama Sequence*. Stop and rest when necessary, pause for a few moments, and join again when you feel ready. Or stop altogether for the day and take up your practice again the next day.

Pranayama #4—Surya and Chandra Bhedana

Surya: sun, solar, heating, right nostril.
Chandra: moon, lunar, cooling, left nostril.
Bhedana: clear, cleanse, free flowing.

Perform this kumbhaka in order to clear the two principal nadis, ida and pingala, also known as the sun (surya, right nostril) and moon (chandra, left nostril), and also to cleanse the overall system of nadis throughout the body.

The solar right side is said to be like the sun: fiery, generating heat and light, active, and masculine. The lunar left side is said to be like the moon: cooling, receptive, dark, moist, and feminine. Through alternate nostril breathing and kumbhaka, and using this pranayama, you aim to balance your solar and lunar energies.

Like bhastrika (the third pranayama), the fourth pranayama offers the possibilitiy of a longer retention because the retention is performed only after inhalation (antara kumbhaka) and not after exhalation. Use vishnu mudra hand position. (See instructions for vishnu mudra hand positioning in the video series, *A Guide to the Pranayama Sequence.*)

Pranayama #5—Sitali

Sitali: cooling.

Sitali is performed on the inhalation by opening the mouth, forming the lips into an "O," extending the tongue out of the mouth, and curling the ends into a funnel shape. Then draw the breath in across the tongue with a sucking noise and perform kumbhaka after completing the inhalation.

Both techniques, ujjayi and sitali, involve narrowing the glottis. This action enables you to stretch, lengthen, and regulate your breath. With sitali you can experience the inhalation as a pull; draw the breath in with a suction-like action, a sipping-in of nectar.

References from The Shiva Samhita

- The when the skillful Yogi, knowing the laws of the action of prana and apana vayus, can drink the air through the contraction of the mouth, in the form of a crow bill, he's entitled to liberation. The wise Yogi, who drinks the ambrosial air, destroys fatigue, decay, old age, and injuries.[1]

- When he drinks the air through the crow-bill, contemplating that it goes to the mouth of the kundalini, diseases of the lungs are cured.[2]

- When the wise Yogi drinks the fluid day and night through the crow-beak, his diseases are destroyed, he acquires the powers of clairaudience and clairvoyance.[3]

---

1   *The Shiva Samhita*   III–70
2   *The Shiva Samhita*   III–74
3   *The Shiva Samhita*   III–75

"If Pranayama is practiced then the diseases present in the body, sense organs, and mind will be cured, allowing the mind to achieve concentration and perceive the inner self."[1]

– Sri K. Pattabhi Jois

---

1 *Yoga Mala* pg 18

Vayu Siddhi

Vayu

Prana is the word in yoga for life energy, the creative force of the universe, the power behind the ever-renewing cycles of manifestation, the secret spark that brings radiance to the infinite parade of coming and going forms of existence. It is said that prana originates in the heart, "adorned with various desires accompanied by past works, that have no beginning and with egoism (ahamkara)."[1] From its different modifications it receives various names. When prana is confined inside the body through yoga techniques it is called vayu.

Vayu is interiorized energy—animated, awakened life force that becomes potent when sealed within the body through the practice of bandhas (internal locks), dhyana (meditation), and pratyahara (sense withdrawal). Vayu is the sum total of prana or energy that makes up the body.

Vayu is found in five regions, or territories, inside the body. They are: prana, apana, samana, vyana, and udana.

They have the following basic qualities:

(1) Prana vayu (expansive, upward, in-breath).
Territory: upper torso between diaphragm and collarbones.

---

1   *The Shiva Samhita* III–2, 3

(2) Apana vayu (contractive, downward, out-breath).
Territory: lower torso from pelvic floor to navel.

(3) Samana vayu (equal).
Territory: mid torso from navel to diaphragm, associated with the solar plexus, seat of digestive fire.

(4) Vyana vayu (pervasive).
Territory: throughout the microcosm (body).

(5) Udana vayu (up-breath).
Territory: from the throat through the top of the head.

Also, vayu means to blow, and is the name of the important vedic god Vayu, the wind god. Vayu is a symbol of the breath and is known as the life breath of the gods. Mythologically, all of existence is said to be contained within the body of a single, colossal person known as Purusa, the Cosmic Man, and Vayu is his breath. Vayu is also known to be an explorer and a wanderer.

Your own breath, like Vayu, is a natural explorer who, if given the opportunity, can wander, roam, investigate, and open up the vast interior psychological and physical spaces within your body. The skillful yogi enjoys the breath's wandering spirit; he heeds the inward call to explore the full extent of his inspiration and expiration and to dwell in the void in the gaps between breaths.

With courage and devotion the yogi learns to breathe in and out freely, with gusto and subtlety, becoming receptive to the full range of the breath's rhythmic sweep. He uses his breath to overcome fear of the unknown places within his body and psyche. He goes to new, unexplored places within himself, and he befriends his shadow, faces and conquers the inner dragons and hears the sound of "the flute of interior time,"[1] the unequaled inner sound of OM.

---

1   *The Kabir Book, translation by Robert Bly* pg 21

The adventurous yogi enjoys following the wanderings of his breath and thus travels throughout the vastness within himself, awakening his consciousness, learning to enjoy the full extent of his body as an inner refuge.

Vayu is a messenger of the gods. Conscious breathing creates inner discernment, gives you access to buddhi—your intuition, your innate wisdom, the knowledge that lives within you awaiting your attention—ever-ready to come into expression. Utilizing the breath as a messenger gives you the power to make rapid and subtle distinctions between grosser, harmful, dead-end directions and intelligent, genuine, fine, and worthy promptings within you. Listening to your breathing helps you refine your overall emotional ability to listen inwardly so that you can receive important messages about how to choose wisely for now and for your future benefit. Without the breath's help this potent innate knowledge living in your depths can remain hidden, dormant within you. And thus the skillful yogi comes to trust his breath as a messenger, a direct channel of his unique, personal wisdom flowing forth from the deep source within his body.

Vayu is known and feared for his power and strength. At times he blows with a ferocity that uproots mountains, trees, houses, and anything else in his way. His formidable strength commands respect but also is a testament to the power of the breath as a main vehicle that carries prana throughout the body. The power of the breath also speaks to its central role in the creative activity of asana and pranayama mastery.

References from The Hatha Yoga Pradipika

- The vayu should be made to enter the shushumna without restraint by him who has practiced control of the breathing and has awakened the kundalini by the fire.[1]

- It (the breath) should be expelled again and filled again and again, just as a pair of bellows of the blacksmith is worked. In the same way the air (vayu) of the body should be moved intelligently. It quickly awakens the kundalini, purifies the system, gives pleasure and is beneficial.[2]

References from The Shiva Samhita

- Contract the perineum and draw the apana vayu upward and join it with samana vayu; bend the prana vayu downward and then let the wise yogi bind them in trinity in the navel. Through this practice, the vayu (life force) enters the middle channel of the shushumna, the body is invigorated by it, the bones are firmly knitted, the heart of the yogi becomes full.[3]

- According to the strength of one's practice in commanding the vayu, he gets command over his body; the wise, remaining in the spirit, enjoys the world in the present body.[4]

- When the Vayu moves through all the nadis, then the fluids of the body get extraordinary force and energy.[5]

- By habitual exercise of contemplating muladhara, one's vayu enters the middle channel (shushumna).[6]

- In the heart there is a brilliant lotus with twelve petals... the prana lives there...[7]

---

1 *The Hatha Yoga Pradipika* IV–19
2 *The Hatha Yoga Pradipika* II–62, 63, 65
3 *The Shiva Samhita* IV–21
4 *The Shiva Samhita* V–41
5 *The Shiva Samhita* V–54
6 *The Shiva Samhita* V–73
7 *The Shiva Samhita* III–1, 2

- From the different modifications of the prana, it receives various names…prana, apana, samana, udana, vyana represent the major five divisions of interior prana called the five vayus.[1]

- The prana and apana vayus are the highest agents…[2]

- The seat of prana vayu is the heart, of apana the anus (of samana, the region about the navel, of udana, the throat, while vyana moves all over the body).[3]

---

1   *The Shiva Samhita*   III–3, 4
2   *The Shiva Samhita*   III–6
3   *The Shiva Samhita*   III–7

Siddhi

Literally perfection, or success, as in one who experiences the
Self and thus attains the highest knowledge. The term siddhi
also means magic powers, superhuman or extraordinary powers,
that result from devotion to practice, and particularly from asana
and pranayama practice. There is a caution in the teachings to
use siddhis for self-realization and not to get caught in merely
enjoying them or using them for lower purposes.

Here are a few examples of siddhis that are helpful in
developing a dynamic, fruitful understanding of pranayama.

Vayu siddhi—Refers to mastery over the flow, movement, and
direction of internal prana, of life force within you. Attaining
vayu siddhi involves undertaking tapas, discipline and sacrifice
in order to purify the nadis, the subtle, pranic channels, and to
set free the prana within you. Pattabhi Jois used to say, "free
breathing you take," because free breathing is the main means
of cleansing the network of nadis so that prana can flow freely
throughout your body. Without pranayama practice the nadi
channels are said to be clogged, impure, obstructed, and thus
success (siddhi) cannot be attained. Success is obtained by
repetitiously and intently following the movement patterns of
inhaling and exhaling. Contemplating the concept of vayu siddhi
reminds you of the extraordinary powers that will come to you
by making a careful study of the energetic vayu patterns that
are associated with breathing. Through illuminating the vayu
patterns of breathing you light up the subtle body; you learn
how to redirect the movements of prana and apana vayus, to
internalize your awareness and cause your prana to withdraw into
the middle channel where the experience of the Void awaits.

Vigraha siddhi—Mastery over the microcosm. Vigraha
siddhi is said to be obtained by performing uddhyana bandha,
a practice that is in constant use in pranayama. As the internal
system of nadis is cleansed and you attain control of over internal

movements of prana, you come to know the inner field of the body. Using your internalized awareness to fully animate your psychic world leads you embrace a more global perspective, as though your personal feeling of "I am" extends to the entire cosmos. You see the entire world as yourself; you love the world as yourself.

Darduri siddhi—The frog jump power. Mula bandha is said to give darduri siddhi, frog leap power. I love this image because it is animal, visual, dynamic, and fun: awakening the pelvic floor will bring incredible buoyancy and leaping power. Through practicing mula bandha you can experience an extra powerful sense of the earth and a corresponding extraordinary lightness, a rebound, a natural counter-response that carries you away from the earth. Imagining darduri siddhi, the ability to resoundingly leap away from the earth, facilitates power, strength, and ease in all variety of jumping, such as jumping back and jumping through in vinyasa transitions.

Samadhi siddhi—Refers to the mastery of the mind, to success in the practice of cognitive absorption. The practice of isvara pranidhana is said to give samadhi siddhi. Isvara pranidhana means inward devotion to the Self, or surrender to Divinity, to the Lord. In pranayama, devotion and surrender form the essential background context that helps balance the willful effort that is required to learn to regulate and control your breathing. Through surrender and devotion you become void-minded; you gain the power to focus your mind, to become wholly, pin-pointedly absorbed in the immediate experience at hand and yet retain a wide, sky-like, spacious mental clarity, a receptivity, a lazy, winking purposelessness that balances the seriousness and intensity of your focused concentration.

"Pranayama means taking the subtle power of the vital wind through rechaka (exhalation), puraka (inhalation) and kumbhaka (retention)."[1]

– Sri K. Pattabhi Jois

---

1   *Yoga Mala* pg 23

Afterword

Darshan: to see, to be seen by God, to behold the sacred, to be blessed by having been looked upon by an auspicious deity.

When visiting an Indian temple, the installed deity is usually located far to the rear of the temple even though you can catch an enticing glimpse of the specially adorned murti (form of the icon) looking out toward you from the recesses of the temple. There is usually a series of rooms, walkways, doors, or curtains that separate the murti from the temple entrance. This spatial separation reminds you that you must cross over a series of thresholds, physical, energetic, and psychic, in order to receive darshan, to arrive at the sacred center, the place of prayer and communion.

Often the crowds are so large and pressing that it can be hot, long, difficult, and bothersome to move through the labyrinth into the heart of the temple to the awaiting icon. Fortunately the place of communion brings relief, a welcome pause. The interior of the temple is refreshingly remote, and ponderously silent. The psychic atmosphere in there sharply contrasts the nearby outer world with its noise, activity, and bustle.

Periodically the priest will perform a small puja (worship) that consists of chanting mantras, offering flowers, and waving a flame in front of the deity. He then offers the purifying flame to you, as well as flowers from the altar, and a sip of the blessed water. Periodically he will draw the set of curtains shut temporarily hiding the deity and himself while he offers some hidden prayers to the deity. You stand with other onlookers prayerfully waiting for the curtains to be drawn open again so that each of you can have darshan, an auspicious moment where you see and are seen by the sacralized murti.

The physical and mental efforts that are required to stop your mind's activity when you suspend the breath in kumbhaka during pranayama practice are what lead you inward across the inner thresholds to reach the silent place of refuge within, the sacred center of your body temple. You arrive in the cave of the heart, and there resides the great source of the breath, an auspicious deity secreted away deep within your inner recesses.

Sometimes this deity, the Self, is described being the size of a thumb, sometimes as having the form of a smokeless, unwavering flame that never burns down, and the light from this flame illuminates the vast cave of the heart. You undertake the ordeal of tapas, of long-term practice, of controlling the breath, to become dynamic enough, still enough, and silent enough to catch a glimpse of this Secret One, the source of the inner flame, the source of the breath.

Saint and Poet Kabir said:

"Friend tell me: 'Who is God?'
'God is the breath inside the breath' "[1]

May you benefit from your devotion to the practice of pranayama; may you withdraw inward, cross each important threshold, dwell in the alive silence and stillness between breaths, become void-minded, attain vayu siddhi, and have darshan with the ever-elusive Secret One.

Enjoy, OM!

---

1   *The Kabir Book, translation by Robert Bly*   pg 33

"Vinyasa means 'breathing and movement system.'"[1]

    – Sri K. Pattabhi Jois

Glossary

Anahata: the unstruck (sound). Fourth chakra, heart center. Home of the in-breath pattern called prana vayu. Center of the region of prana vayu which spans the upper chest cavity from the diaphragm to the collarbones.

References from The Hatha Yoga Pradipika

- ...Sitting in Padmasana, he should hear anahata, the unstruck sound, attentively.[1]

- ...When the body becomes lean, the face glows with delight, anahata nada manifests, and eyes are clear, body is healthy, bindu under control, and appetite (for simple, healthy food) increases, then one should know that the nadis are purified and success in hatha yoga is approaching.[2]

Antara Kumbhaka: antara (internal); kumbhaka (retention). To retain the breath after inhalation. (See entry for **Kumbhaka**.)

Bahya Kumbhaka: bahya (external); kumbhaka (retention). To retain the breath after exhalation. (See entry for **Kumbhaka**.)

Bandha: bind; bond; arrest; capture; put together; lock; shut; close; redirect; seal; stop; cohere. Bandhas come under the

---

1 *The Hatha Yoga Pradipika* II–15
2 *The Hatha Yoga Pradipika* II–78

broad category of mudra (seal) and their usage is one of the most important foundational techniques used in the practice of ashtanga yoga. There are three main bandhas: mula bandha (root lock, pelvic floor, first or root chakra), uddhyana bandha (flying up, stomach lock, second chakra), and jalandhara bandha (chin lock, fifth or throat chakra).

A bandha is a set of muscular contractions in a specific area of the body that serves to stop and redirect the flow of prana (energy, or life force) within the body. Applying bandhas involves sealing in one's life force to direct, purify, and unblock the flow of energy within the vast network of pranic channels throughout the body. Skillfully locking specific locations along the central axis enables the yogi to confine his prana in the middle so that he can untie the powerful knots of ignorance that are formed by his karma and conditioned habit patterns. The sacred texts say that "like a man and his shadow go together, so too do the prana (life force) and the atma (Self within the body)."[1] Thus the yogi utilizes bandhas to train his mind onto the movements of his prana, and he improves his chances of glimpsing the elusive Self who "runs swifter than thought and yet never moves."[2]

References from The Hatha Yoga Pradipika
- In order to awaken this goddess, who is sleeping at the entrance of the great door (brahma dwara) mula bandha, uddhyana bandha, jalandhara bandha should be performed.[3]

Dhyana: from Sanskrit for meditation, the seventh of the eight limbs of Patanjali's *Yoga Sutras*, aimed at self-realization and self-knowledge. When the mind is no longer distracted from the object of concentration, then dhyana is realized. Dhyana is also:

(1) A general word used in many sacred texts meaning intense

---

1 *Prasnopanishad (The Prasna Upanishad)* Query III–3

2 *The Upanishads, Breath of The Eternal* pg 27

3 *The Hatha Yoga Pradipika* III–5

focus, concentration, awareness, meditation, or
even samadhi.

(2) One of the foundational techniques used in ashtanga yoga as
put forth by Sri K. Pattabhi Jois in his book *Yoga Mala*.

References from The Hatha Yoga Pradipika
- So long as the breath is restrained in the body, so long as the
  mind is undisturbed, and so long as the gaze is fixed between
  the eyebrow, there is no fear of death.[1]

- Steadiness of mind comes when the air moves freely in the
  middle. (That is the manonmani condition, which is attained
  when the mind becomes calm.)[2]

Khecari: one who moves in Kha, the void within the heart.
Kha: void, space, emptiness.
Cara: moves in, walks in, vehicle of.

Literally "the one who moves in Kha, the Void." Khecari mudra
refers to the practice technique of withdrawing awareness into the
root of the palate area just above the mouth and below the brain
along the central axis.

Using khecari, the void-minded yogi is pulled inward. The
mouth becomes an uncluttered, sacred cave, an inner temple
spot, a power place, a seat of focused awareness, a primary source
of kinesthetic intelligence and meditation. (Find more on khecari
in the "Mudras" section on page 76 of this book.)

Kumbhaka: retention or suspension of breath ("pot-like").
Phase between puraka (inhalation) and/or rechaka (exhalation).

References from the Hatha Yoga Pradipika
- So long as the (breathing) air stays in the body, it is called life.
  Death consists in the passing out of the (breathing) air. It is
  therefore necessary to restrain the breath.[3]

---

1 *The Hatha Yoga Pradipika* II–40
2 *The Hatha Yoga Pradipika* II–42
3 *The Hatha Yoga Pradipika* II–3

- Respiration being disturbed, the mind becomes disturbed. By restraining respiration, the yogi gets steadiness of mind.[1]

- Kundalini awakens by kumbhaka, and by its awakening, shushumna becomes free from impurities.[2]

- On the completion of kumbhaka, the mind should be given rest.[3]

- Kumbhaka is the keeping of the air confined inside.[4]

Muladhara: root or earth support.

Mula: earth, root, foundation.

Dhara: support.

Location: lower pelvic region.

Description: red lotus flower; four petals; resting place for dormant kundalini shakti; origin of shushumna nadi; location of mula bandha.

Muladhara is the first of the seven major chakras (wheels or lotuses) that are arranged along the most glorious vertical axis. Muladhara is the foundational chakra, the one location and the best image to support the yogi in learning the visual language of classic hatha yoga as is found in the sacred texts.

References from The Shiva Samhita

- The practitioner of pranayama ought always to meditate upon muladhara…[5]

- Let one thus meditates daily, without negligence, on his own swayambhu linga (muladhara); and have no doubts that from this will come all powers as he conquers the mind and restrains his breath and life force.[6]

---

1   *The Hatha Yoga Pradipika*   II–2
2   *The Hatha Yoga Pradipika*   II–75
3   *The Hatha Yoga Pradipika*   II–77
4   *The Hatha Yoga Pradipika*   II–45
5   *The Shiva Samhita*   V–68
6   *The Shiva Samhita*   V–68

- Inside the lower pelvis, "two digits above the rectum and two digits below the organ is the adhara lotus, having a dimension of four digits."[1]

- In the pericarp of the adhara lotus, there is the triangular, beautiful yoni (force center, symbol of the female organ), hidden and kept secret in all the tantras (yogic texts). In it is the supreme goddess Kundalini of the form of electricity in a coil. It has three coils and a half (like a serpent) and rests there at the mouth of shushumna. It represents the creative force of the world (and also represents the source of your creative force) and is always engaged in creation.[2]

- Two fingers above the rectum and two fingers below the linga, four fingers in width is a space (with a shape) like a bulbous root. Within this space is the yoni (force center symbolized by the female organ) having its face toward the back; that space is called the root, there dwells the goddess Kundalini. She has three and a half coils and catching her tail in her own mouth rests in the hole of shushumna.[3]

- The wise man who always contemplates on this muladhara obtains the darduri siddhi, the frog jump power![4]

Nadi: hollow tube or channel; vessel. Nadis are part of the most basic tantric and hatha yoga imagery and can be thought of as invisible, esoteric nerve channels that carry prana or fine energy throughout the subtle energetic body (pranamaya kosha). The nadis conduct prana via a vast network of pranic channels that branch and spread throughout the entire body. The nadis also coalesce toward the center, joining into larger, individually named nadis at the body's core, culminating with shushumna (most glorious) nadi, the largest and most important nadi.

1   *The Shiva Samhita* II–21
2   *The Shiva Samhita* II–22, 23, 24
3   *The Shiva Samhita* V–56, 57
4   *The Shiva Samhita* V–64

References from the Hatha Yoga Pradipika
- When the system of nadis becomes clear of the impurities by controlling the prana, the air (vayu), piercing the entrance of the shushumna, enters it easily.[1]

References from The Shiva Samhita:
- The nadi called ida is on the left side, coiling round the shushumna; it goes to the right nostril.[2]

- These nadis are spread through the body crosswise and lengthwise; they are the vehicles of sensation...(and keep watch over the movements of vayu [interior prana, air]; they regulate motor functions as well).[3]

- The nadi called pingala is on the right side, coiling around the central vessel; it enters the left nostril.[4]

- The nadi which is between ida and pingala is certainly shushumna—it has six stages, six forces, six lotuses, six chakras known to yogis.[5]

Pranayama: breath control.
Prana: life force, energy, or Shakti; sacralized energy.
Yama: restraint, death, bind.
Ayama: the opposite of restraint, or to unbind.

The fourth limb of Patanjali's ashtanga (eight limbs) in *The Yoga Sutras*. A technique within hatha yoga practice that utilizes breath retention in various capacities in order internalize the awareness of the breath so that prana, life force, can awaken and go up the central pranic channel from the yoni (fountain, source) at the base, to sahasra, the magnificent lotus at the crown.

---

1 *The Hatha Yoga Pradipika* II–41
2 *The Shiva Samhita* II–25
3 *The Shiva Samhita* II–31
4 *The Shiva Samhita* II–26
5 *The Shiva Samhita* II–27

Pranayama practice helps the yogi to consecrate the internal, sacred temple of the body called "Brahmanda" microcosm.

Some descriptions of pranayama include:
- free breathing
- internalized breath
- balanced breath
- breath control
- unrestrained life energy
- prana siddhi—perfection of prana
- prana vidya—knowledge of energy (prana), knowledge of the subtle body
- vayu siddhi—power over the five vayus

Puraka: the term for inhalation used in pranayama

Rechaka: expulsion. The term for exhalation used in pranayama. During rechaka "The air should be expelled slowly and not violently."[1]

Sahasra: thousand-petaled or thousand-spoked. The seventh and final major chakra whose location is at or just above the crown of the head. Sahasra is the highest point along the pillar of light that is shushumna. It is the peak of Mount Meru, or world mountain, that corresponds to the spinal column and to the central axis.

Siddhi: mastery or perfection of yoga techniques and the powers that you win from such mastery. To acquire siddhis, or powers, is one reason to yoke yourself to a daily ashtanga practice. (Read more on page 120.)

Shushumna: most glorious. Shushumna is one of the many names for the central and foremost nadi, or pranic channel, that spans the vertical axis within the core of the body between the pelvic floor and the crown of the head. Shushumna is the conduit

---

1   *The Hatha Yoga Pradipika* III–11, 12

for carrying awakened shakti—the coiled, serpentine, goddess energy—from the depths upward to the symbolic thousand-petaled lotus at the crown of the head.

Vayu: to blow. Prana (life force) is called vayu inside the body. Vayu is divided into five territories within the body. Each of the five vayus serve as the governor, a regulator of prana, within a given area of the body. The five vayus are prana, apana, samana, vyana, and udana.

Vayu is also the ancient vedic wind god; he represents a deification of the element air or wind. The stories and hymns devoted to the breath (as Vayu) establish the idea that the act of breathing is not only physically essential, but equally essential is that breathing helps the yogi realize his spiritual nature. (Read more on page 115.)

Viloma: viloma is the second most basic pranayama technique after ujjayi and involves stopping or interrupting the inhalation or exhalation in a set of stages. The word viloma literally means against the hair, as in when you rub a cat's fur the wrong way, and derives its name from the immediate prickly reaction that naturally results when you interrupt your breathing. To perform viloma you interrupt either the inhalation or exhalation with a series of pauses or gaps. During the gaps you stop and retain the breath for a few seconds. You will find several viloma exercises presented in the video series, *A Guide to Ujjayi Breathing*. The exercises can emphasize working with extending the breath and thus have shorter retentions, or they can emphasize retention and thus have longer intervals during the gaps. All the exercises have three interruptions; the more difficult ones include longer kumbhakas (retentions) after the final pause when the lungs are either completely full or completely empty.

Yoni: place of birth; source; origin; spring; fountain; place of rest; repository; receptacle; seat; abode; home; lair; nest; stable.

Yoni covers a range of meanings all describing the temple floor within muladhara at the pelvic base, the home and resting place of the coiled animal within. Through the sacrificial fire of awareness cultivated during yoga practice, the goddess energy known as Shakti—the animator of the inner world; she who gives birth; bringer of ideas, imagination, and consciousness—awakens and takes center stage. The word yoni helps map shushumna and provides helpful, descriptive imagery for how to orient yourself devotionally in asana and pranayama practice.

References

Translated by, Pancham Sinh, *The Hatha Yoga Pradipika* (New Delhi, India: Munshiram Manoharlal Publishers Pvt. Ltd., 2001).

Translated by, S.C. Vasu, *The Yoga Samhita* (Delhi, India: Sri Satguru Publications, Indological and Oriental Publishers, 2005).

Translated by, Swami Venkatesananda, *The Supreme Yoga, Yoga Vasistha* (Delhi, India: Motilal Banarsidass Publishers Pvt. Ltd., 2006).

Translated by, Robert Bly, *The Kabir Book* (Boston, USA: A Seventies Press Book, Beacon Press, 1977).

Translated by, Swami Prabhavananda and Frederick Manchester, *The Upanishads, Breath of The Eternal* (New York, USA: New American Library, a division of Penguin Putnam Inc., 2002).

Translated by Coleman Barks, *The Essential Rumi* (New York, USA: HarperCollins Publishers, 2004).

Translated by, Swami Chinmayananda, *Prasnopanisad* (Mumbai, India: Central Chinmaya Mission Trust, 2002).

Sri K. Pattabhi Jois, *Yoga Mala* (New York, USA: North Point Press, 2002).

Vyass Houston M.A., *The Yoga Sutra Workbook, The Certainty of Freedom* (Warwick, USA: American Sanskrit Institute, 1995).

B.K.S. Iyengar, Light on the Yoga Sutras of Patanjali (Uttar Pradesh, India: HarperCollins Publishers, 2010

Bad Man

Sri K. Pattabhi Jois (Guruji) demanded that his students follow his method with clear and strict accuracy, but he achieved this partly by tolerance, understanding, smiles, hugs and overall benevolence. He could be stern and uncompromising but also understanding and respectful of individual difference. When you bent or broke the rules he jestingly or punitively called you "bad man" or "bad lady" depending on whether you acted out of negligence or in service of expressing your individuality within the confines of the system.

By calling you "bad man," Guruji was perhaps chastising you for not respecting the rules of the system thus reminding you of the importance of those rules. And he was also perhaps showing you with humor that he understood that learning yoga requires individuality, for you to be yourself in a basic, fundamental way. One time a student became offended when he called her bad lady. He smiled and chuckled and said, "bad means good."

His teaching reflected the notion that following each rule every time is not always in the best overall service of gaining yoga knowledge. But neither is disregarding the rules too liberally or too often. Guruji understood that two contradictory conditions need to coexist for a yoga lineage to be effective in continuing to pass down knowledge between generations. First, a lineage needs to be respected and valued, and thus carefully upheld by each student. Second, each student also needs to have the freedom to bend or even break the rules at certain times. In either case a student needs a high degree of inner-trust, to have the self-confidence and receptivity to explore yoga's possibilities for himself.

Guruji himself walked a different and individual path throughout his life. He left his family and village by his own decision to learn yoga from his Guru. He and his wife chose each other in a "love" marriage. And he fearlessly pioneered his fiery, different, new yoga method. He thoroughly understood the necessity of being a "bad man," of stepping off the prescribed path, taking control of his own life, and making the choices that he felt would give him the best chance for success.

The development of yoga through the generations depends on the person who has the daring and confidence to go into the unknown and find the unique, though universal, knowledge within himself. Each authentic yogi has to be a "bad man" or "bad lady," he or she has to walk the edge between respect for what came before and curiosity for the new, the unknown, the unique and the solitary. Ultimately following a lineage and attaining success in yoga requires attaining self-knowledge through consulting the heart, refining and clarifying intention, lastingly appreciating the teachings that have been received, and finding kindred spirits along the path.